The Liver Doctor

The Liver Doctor

Stories of Love, Loss and Regeneration

DR CYRIAC ABBY PHILIPS

HARPER NON-FICTION

First published in India by Harper Non-Fiction 2026
An imprint of HarperCollins *Publishers*
HarperCollins *Publishers* India, Cyber City,
Building 10-A, Gurugram, Haryana – 122002, India
www.harpercollins.co.in

2 4 6 8 10 9 7 5 3 1

P-ISBN: 978-93-6569-523-6
E-ISBN: 978-93-6569-908-1

Typeset in 11.25 pt/14.8 Arno Pro
by HarperCollins *Publishers* India Pvt. Ltd

Printed and bound in
India by Manipal Technologies Limited

FSC www.fsc.org MIX Paper | Supporting responsible forestry FSC™ C043100

This book is produced from independently certified FSC® paper to ensure responsible forest management.

HarperCollins *Publishers*, Macken House, 39/40 Mayor Street Upper, Dublin 1, D01 C9W8, Ireland

For

My patients, past, present and future, because you teach me the medicine that I need to learn and not be taught.

Doctors, past, present and future, because you alone stand between life and death, fighting against your infirmity for strangers you consider family so that they may be with theirs.

My wife, Teena, because the deepest love is always carried in sights, sometimes left unsaid and at times penned.

My children, Alanna, Aideen and Arthur, because when I am gone, all the love in here is yours, and yours only.

The detailed notes pertaining to this book are available on the HarperCollins *Publishers* India website. Scan this QR code to access the same.

Contents

Preface

FOR MANY OF YOU WHO KNOW ME—OR HAVE HEARD OF ME—it may come as a surprise that I never originally dreamt of becoming a doctor. Life, with its own mysterious design, led me down this path, and today I have no regrets. In writing this book, two very different worlds collided. On one side is my everyday life as a doctor: I care deeply for my patients and their families, even though the weight of our shared struggles sometimes pulls me into dark places and affects my mental well-being—something I never truly understood before stepping into this profession. When HarperCollins India first approached me with a book proposal, it felt as though I was being drawn back to a long-forgotten part of myself—the other world; a time when I would weave stories to fend off loneliness and fear. As a child, I was haunted by solitude and darkness, and invented characters to keep me company. Those stories, born out of necessity, set me free. In this book, I merge the raw, real-life experiences of my medical practice with that childhood love for storytelling, presenting them in a way I hope everyone can understand.

To be completely honest, I chose medicine partly because I was never very good at math. Yet, even as I immersed myself in the often-ordinary routines of clinical work, my passion for storytelling never faded. In fact, practising medicine opened my eyes to a world of reality that was richer and more complex than I had ever imagined. From my early training in medicine and surgery, through a focused study in internal medicine, and finally in my specialization in hepatology—the branch that deals with the study of the liver—I have collected countless stories. These tales come from patients and their families: stories of survival and of loss, filled with unforgettable memories, deep wounds and scars that have quietly taken residence in a corner of my heart. All these experiences built up inside me, demanding to be shared—a lesson to be taught, a truth to be learnt, a feeling that simply could not remain silent. I longed to bring you along, yet the demands of being a clinical doctor meant that I was often confined to outpatient clinics and hospital corridors, where the practice of medicine threatened to consume every moment of my life.

Then came Twitter. My journey into social media began simply enough—catching up with friends and sharing family photos on platforms like Orkut, Facebook and Instagram. One day, I discovered Twitter, and it surprised me with its power to change public perception, spark meaningful dialogues and draw attention to important issues. My first encounter with it was not entirely pleasant. I used to admire the credibility of those blue-tick verified accounts—especially the medical and health profiles—and I was already deep into research on alcohol-related liver disease and injuries caused by drugs and herbs. I started with my original handle, @drabbyphilips, hoping to share important insights about liver injuries and the risks of alternative medicines. However, instead of focusing on the message, many began to fixate on me. The internet can be harsh, and soon I was mislabelled—a Christian missionary; a priest-abused, mentally troubled, big-pharma endorser; and even an anti-Hindu communist from Kerala—simply because I was discussing studies on Ayurvedic therapies, a traditional treatment method with roots in India, also called 'Hindu Medicine' by the British. Overwhelmed by trolling, abuse and harassment, I lost my way. I stepped back, continued my work, strengthened my research and learnt how to publish solid evidence. When I returned to Twitter, I found that while the platform had not changed, the way I communicated with its often-harsh crowd had. I began to share the stories of my patients and their families—not just from my point of view, but by embracing their voices as well. These were more than just anecdotes; they became lessons, fresh ways of learning, and a window into the world of hepatology and clinical medicine seen through empathy, care and even the bittersweet pain that accompanies our struggles. The stories ranged from herbal liver injuries to rare liver diseases, drug-induced injuries, the effects of alcohol, challenging diagnoses and exhausting battles fought within hospital walls—sometimes ending in the loss of a patient. They told of not only the physical challenges faced by patients but also the heartbreaking journeys of their families and the deep, unseen scars left on the hearts of those who treated them.

Beyond the science, this book is a tribute to the essential qualities of medical care that are becoming rare today: humanism, evidence-based practice and empathy. It reveals how the process of caring for patients with liver disease—marked by hope, heartbreak and resilience—not only transforms the lives of those who suffer but also deeply affects the doctors who treat them. I share these stories not just to inform, but to remind you of the enduring strength and compassion that lies at the heart of medicine.

One story, first written online in May 2022—the very one that opens this book—went viral after I posted it on Twitter. It reached 2 million impressions, received 82,300 likes and was retweeted 43,100 times. It was published by Oxford Medical and even featured on Der Spiegel's influential podcast series, *Ein rätselhafter Patient.* I never anticipated such a reaction, nor did I expect my role as a clinician to transform so dramatically. That single story changed the way I saw my work: I began to view my profession not merely as one of prescribing treatments but also as one of teaching. After all, one of the true meanings of being a doctor is to *teach*. From that point on, my Twitter presence evolved. I became known as The Liver Doc, with my handle shifting to @theliverdr. More stories followed—long-form threads that amassed tens of millions of views, turning into a new format for medical education that drew interest first from India and later from audiences around the globe. In just a few years, my account grew to become the largest medical handle on Twitter in India.

This book is an ambitious, original work that brings together my personal experiences treating patients with liver diseases in a way that is both educational and deeply human. Each chapter breaks down a specific condition (or conditions), explains the challenges of diagnosing it, and shares historical insights, fascinating mythological references and treatment options drawn from years of clinical experience that will enrich and inform.

At the heart of every story is an exploration of the liver—a uniquely resilient organ that manages to regenerate even under tremendous strain. I must admit that I have altered names, genders, ages and other personal details, as well as the time and place of events, to protect the privacy of my patients and their families—except in cases where the information was already public. Every detail is supported by evidence from published literature, as shown by the more than 500 citations listed at the end of this book.

This book is meant for everyone: patients, their families, healthcare workers and anyone interested in understanding the profound impact of liver disease. It offers a clear window into the latest clinical studies, innovative treatments like liver dialysis and healthy donor stool transplants, and even unexpected advances in liver transplantation procedures.

I invite you to join me on this journey—a journey that is as much about science as it is about life, hope and the relentless pursuit of healing. This is a book you won't just read; it is a book you'll experience, one that will leave you better informed, more compassionate and ready to engage with the complex world of liver health. I hope you enjoy reading these pages as much as I enjoyed writing them. I wrote this book for healthcare workers, so they can learn, dream and care with deeper understanding. I wrote it for you and your family, so that you can know when to fight and when to let go. For my patients who died, to show you how bravely they fought and how their families stood by them. For you, the reader, to show that doctors are human too—filled with fears, doubts and hopes about life, death and disease. I wrote it for both current and future patients, to remind you that true medical science is deeply caring. I wrote it for myself because I want to make peace with what I have lost and what I will lose in the future. And I wrote it for my family, so that they may know how I fought ... how we fought ... and how it all ends.

I never wanted to become a doctor.
I always wanted to write and tell stories.

I am a liver doctor.
I have no regrets about becoming one.

In this book, you will see both worlds collide.

Cyriac Abby Philips
(The Liver Doc)

Kochi, Kerala

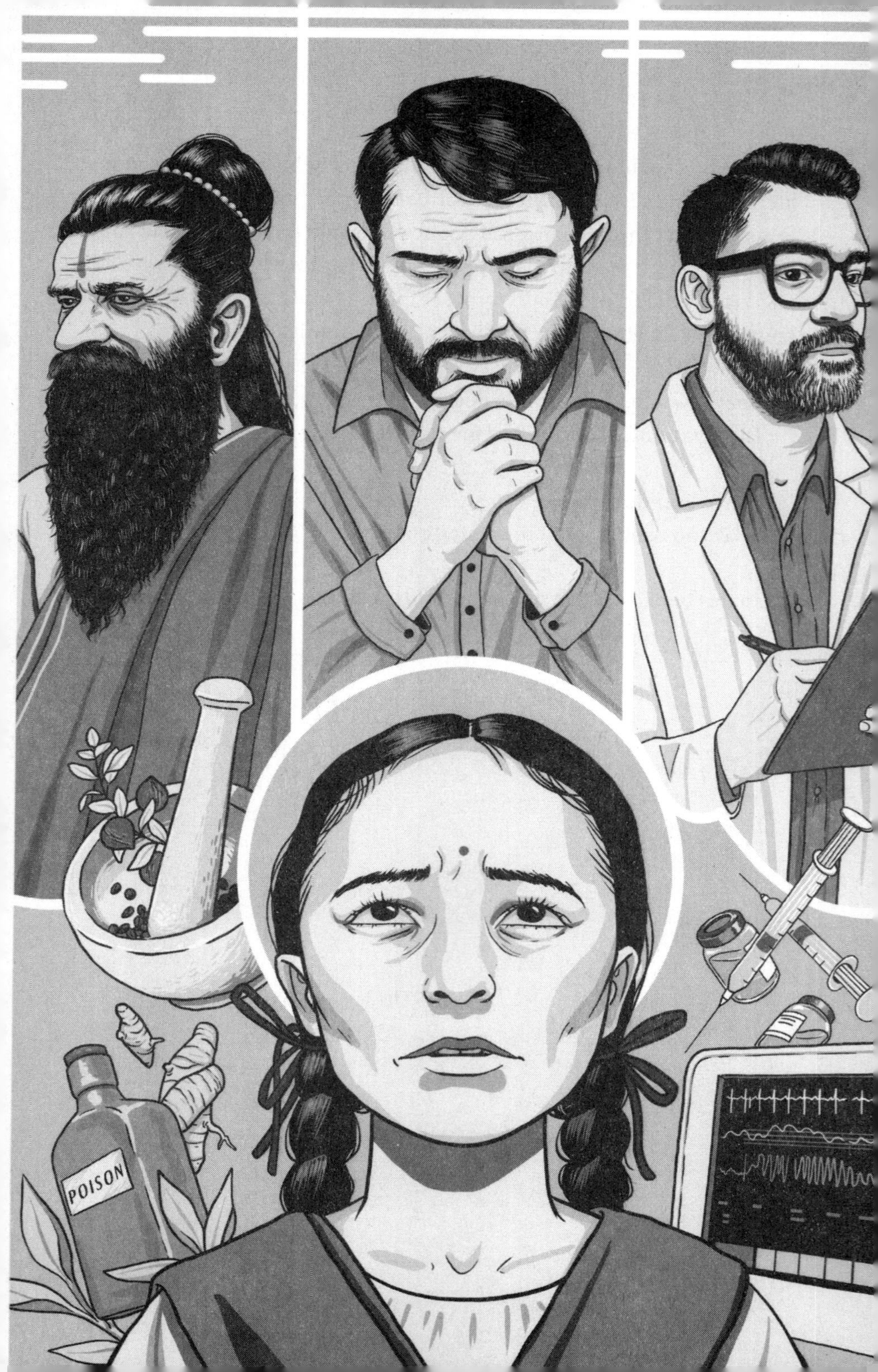
POISON

Prologue
Jesus's Miracle, Krishna's War

The Little Girl in the Woods

'Where the art of medicine is loved, there is also love for humanity.'
—HIPPOCRATES

Love

OBSERVE. LOOK CLOSELY. DO YOU SEE IT?

From the time you are born, everything is going away from you. Your first friend, your best friend, your first kiss, your last. Parents, beloved family, children. First pet, and the ones that come after. Your whole life is slowly floating away, one day at a time.

Except for Death.

From the time you are born, Death becomes your friend. The only one destined to advance towards you and finally embrace you. Death is your friend. Always has been.

When everyone else is moving away, Death is there, waiting for you.

Why did I want to become a doctor, knowing that Death would always be part of the job? Doctors are the unexpected, graceful redeemers within

Death's design—a process, whether swift or slow, that strips people down into patients or hollow shells of who they once used to be. I became a doctor not to help people cheat Death but to prepare them to understand *it* and, in the process, learn the value of embracing *life*.

Through sickness and death, this made absolute sense until it became about a child.

It was November 2017. A day like any other. I was waiting for a patient and his family to exit my outpatient room before the next in line came in. Halfway through their exit, a middle-aged man rushed in with a young girl. She was fourteen years old, profoundly jaundiced and lethargic. Even before I could ask them to sit and give me the girl's clinical history, her father, teary-eyed, requested only one thing: 'She has been advised to undergo a liver transplant to prolong her life. We are poor. Can you please help us avoid it?'

Death. Coming for a child. They could not afford a liver transplant, and without it the child was going to die. My heart raced and palms sweated as I looked at the girl, then at her defenceless father and braced myself for the worst case I had ever seen as I got pitted against Death itself.

Saikrishna was well until two months before, when she started feeling lethargic. Typically an active, studious girl, now she just wanted to lie down and not go to school. Once a bright student, her concentration dwindled. She started losing her appetite and slight tremors in both hands made it difficult for her to cope with schoolwork.

Her parents started to notice certain other things as well. Their child was getting darker and thinner. Then came something no one expected: her skin and the whites of her eyes became yellow. Her urine, too, turned a deep yellow. The signs pointed to jaundice.

Jaundice—a sinister symptom of an underlying disease, most often liver-related—is an ancient dread, the earliest records of which can be found on Mesopotamian clay tablets and in the Old Testament. Physicians during Hippocrates's time considered jaundice, like fever, an independent disease, and not just a symptom of an underlying illness.

Saikrishna's parents took her to a nearby multispeciality hospital. Without haste, the doctors started looking aggressively into the underlying cause of her jaundice. Every physician initially looks for common culprits: alcohol use, viral infections and prescription drug use. Alcohol use was effectively ruled out. Next came tests for infectious causes of hepatitis (inflammation of the liver leading to swollen liver cells that eventually die out), such as the hepatitis A, B, C and E viruses. These results came back as negative. The treating doctors then found something strange.

The level of copper in Saikrishna's urine was relatively high. Based on this finding, they started looking for other clues and found that the level of a particular protein in the blood, ceruloplasmin, was low. The ceruloplasmin protein is made inside the liver, and it's responsible for the storing and ferrying of copper to needy tissues. In a genetic condition called Wilson's disease—named after the American-born British neurologist Samuel Alexander Kinnier Wilson, who initially described it in 1912—a mutation in a liver-specific gene called ATP7B results in obstacles to copper transportation within liver cells. This is followed by copper accumulation inside the liver and overflow of excessive copper into the bloodstream, which travels all over the body. The excess copper gets deposited in the brain, eyes and kidneys, leading to organ damage, and any excess is excreted into the urine. As copper transportation fails at the liver-cell level, ceruloplasmin levels go extremely low in persons with Wilson's disease. In Saikrishna's case, the excess copper in the urine and the mildly low ceruloplasmin level made the doctors comfortable enough to diagnose her with Wilson's disease. They started her on various treatments that help bind excess copper and reduce metal toxicity in the body—called chelation therapy.

When Dr Samuel Wilson initially described Wilson's disease, he called it 'hepato-lenticular degeneration', telling of a mysterious illness that mainly affected a specific part of the brain (the lenticular region of the basal ganglia) and the liver. In young people, the resulting insufferable symptoms included psychosis, depression, lack of concentration and tremors, untidy handwriting, excessive salivation, gaping mouth and stiffening muscles. Affected patients either became bed-bound because of progressive brain dysfunction or died a slow and unpleasant death due to liver failure.

It was only three decades later that Professor John Cumings discovered an excess of copper in the brain and liver as the cause of Wilson's disease. He then suggested that to treat it successfully, one must reduce copper levels in the body by chelating (binding metals) it out of the body. In 1951, he found a strange compound that was able to do this. Fearing that the fascist Adolf Hitler would use arsenic-based chemical warfare, researchers at the biochemistry department of the University of Oxford had developed an antidote called dimercaprol that could bind arsenical chemical gas (called lewisite). They named it BAL, for British anti-lewisite. Professors Cumings in London and Denny Brown in Boston independently used BAL to treat Wilson's disease patients and found that they improved! However, there was an issue: BAL actions were short-lived. Multiple injections of the oil-based drug formulation had to be used, which resulted in excruciating pain at injection sites, lessening benefits with repeated administration and several severe side effects. The search for a new chelating agent began.

On a routine day, also in 1951, Charles Dent, a professor studying human metabolism at the University College, London, found that the urine collected from a patient who underwent the removal of part of the liver with a tumour contained a peculiar compound, previously undescribed.

But where did this compound come from? Professor Dent wondered.

A rigorous search of the patient's clinical notes showed that the surgeons had treated the patient with a penicillin antibiotic to prevent infection post-surgery. Two years later, during a self-experimentation, Dr John Michael Walshe at the same university injected himself with a hefty dose of penicillin and found that he excreted the same compound in his urine. The compound was penicillamine.

Dr Walshe soon forgot about this finding and then moved to the US to work in Dr Charles Davidson's liver unit at Harvard Medical School.

One day, a colleague approached Dr Davidson to see about the further management of a patient with Wilson's disease who was now in a terrible state and not responding to repeated doses of BAL. There was nothing more to be done for the patient, and they offered the best supportive care. However, this patient and his hellish plight bothered Dr Walshe. His mind bounced back to that day in London when he had discovered penicillamine in his urine. He thought deeply and remembered that penicillamine may help bind copper. With the help of Dr Davidson, Walshe got 2 grams of pure penicillamine from Professor John Sheehan at the Massachusetts Institute of Technology.

But was penicillamine safe to use?

Dr Walshe remembered the words of a senior colleague from the University College, London. 'Never give an untried compound to a patient that you are not prepared to take yourself,' Professor Charles Dent, who discovered penicillamine, had said.

Medical practice during the bygone era was intensely patient-centric. There were no ethical committees to oversee doctors and researchers because, unlike today's healthcare practice, every experiment and expected clinical outcome was inherently done to improve the patient's life. It was a beautiful war against ailments.

So, without haste, Dr Walshe ingested 1,000 mg of penicillamine to see if anything unusual happened to him. And nothing did. So he gave the rest of the penicillamine to the unwell patient they had previously seen. Notably, the patient excreted copious amounts of copper in the urine. The chelation was working. More experiments and studies later, a stable, less toxic form of penicillamine called D-penicillamine was prepared with the help of multiple pharmaceutical companies. It would become the life-saving, core medicine for patients suffering from Wilson's disease, liberating them from the slow and progressive descent into hell.

It was the same D-penicillamine that Saikrishna received as the frontline defence against her progressive liver failure. However, a few weeks into the treatment, the young girl's liver tests worsened.

What was happening?

Everything was done per the book and protocol, but the response was deviant. The doctors recommended more tests and further admission. Saikrishna's clinical worsening was overwhelming. The girl's father, Manoj, could not take this anymore. Money was being spent, but there were no results, and it was only a matter of time before both money and time ran out.

So he opted for a second opinion.

Saikrishna, who was getting sicker, was taken to another specialist hospital miles away for expert evaluation. Doctors at the second hospital reviewed her medical records. By now, the little girl's appetite was burnt out and she was thinner. The doctors at the new hospital undertook special blood tests to see if the other group had missed any details the first time.

This time, the doctors found something far more sinister than Wilson's disease. A particular test, known as antinuclear antibody, or ANA, was positive in Saikrishna.

~

Antinuclear antibody is an autoantibody seen in specific disease conditions. Autoantibodies are a group of proteins produced by a person's immune system that attack cells or tissues that are part of the person's body. They are akin to a defence mechanism that goes haywire, unable to identify and neutralize the enemy but instead destroying the body's own 'fortress'—a condition called autoimmunity.

In 1948, with the advent of new tests, scientists discovered ANA and found that it was strongly associated with immune-dysfunction-related diseases. In the early 1950s, a Swedish doctor of internal medicine, Jan Gosta Waldenstrom, and an American immunologist, Henry George

Kunkel, noted a strange form of hepatitis (liver inflammation) among young women. This hepatitis lasted very long (a chronic condition), with ups and downs on liver tests, and was associated with an increased fraction of a particular protein in the blood known as gamma globulin (also called hypergammaglobulinemia). These young girls had other clinical features such as joint pains (arthralgia), joint inflammation (arthritis), and sometimes skin rashes and general debility. They came to be known as 'Kunkel Girls' and their disease as 'chronic active hepatitis'. Before long, patients with chronic active hepatitis were being reported worldwide. Multiple researchers from around the globe started looking at associations. They found that autoimmunity, the body's 'immune hit job on itself', identified on crude tests available at the time, was positive in young women with unknown chronic hepatitis.

Years later, in 1962–63, doctors Ian Reay Mackay and Eric John Holborow found that ANA was increasingly detected in young women with chronic active hepatitis, and the term 'autoimmune hepatitis' came into being. Subsequently, ANA detection became central to the diagnosis of autoimmune hepatitis. Once the reason for chronic active hepatitis was apparent and was considered an autoimmune phenomenon, treatment options became clear: anti-immune therapies, of which the most effective and readily available was the use of steroids. The protocol Professor Mackay devised for treating autoimmune hepatitis with steroids remains the cornerstone for treating this dreadful disease, which has taken the lives of many young women in the past.

~

In Saikrishna's case, the high levels of gamma globulin proteins, specifically the immunoglobulin G antibodies produced by a blood cell called a plasma cell, were also high. This, along with ANA, was highly suggestive of autoimmune hepatitis. The autoantibodies were damaging her liver, and steroids were the answer. To confirm autoimmune hepatitis, a liver biopsy was required. Nevertheless, the doctors started Saikrishna on steroid injections to reduce liver inflammation and curb autoimmune damage, as the girl was getting sicker and they were running out of time. As per guideline recommendations, the doctors also added another immunosuppressive drug, azathioprine, to help reduce steroid doses in the long term. Five days after the dual therapy, the young girl's jaundice started reducing, and there was a glimmer of hope. It was a relief that a diagnosis was nigh, and a treatment would improve Saikrishna's rare but difficult-to-diagnose condition. Medical science was winning.

Loss

However, the win was short-lived. A week later, everything turned head over heels. Not only was the jaundice worsening, but the total bilirubin—which reflects the severity of jaundice—peaked at 26 mg/dL (normal levels range from 0.1–1.2 mg/dL). She started developing another menacing complication of liver disease: ascites, the collection of fluid inside the abdomen. It has been known since antiquity under the common name 'dropsy'.

Dropsy has been described in the Papyrus Ebers in ancient Egypt in 1550 BCE and the Atharva Veda, the source of Ayurvedic texts from ancient India, in 1500–1300 BCE; in the latter it was described as 'jalodara'. Hippocrates, the Father of Medicine, described a fearsome outcome in those who developed ascites: 'When the liver is filled with water and bursts into the cavity—the belly is filled with water, and the patient dies.' This was precisely why the doctors feared for Saikrishna. Her liver was failing, and the only thing left to do was offer a life-saving liver transplant.

Distraught at this treatment option, Manoj saw his family and their simple but satisfying life crumble before his eyes. A liver transplant in a country like India is an expensive affair. There is no centralized social security and health insurance system, and patients have to pay out of their own pockets to sustain their right to health. A liver transplant would easily cost around ₹25 lakh (approximately $27,000). Manoj had to beg, borrow or steal to make it happen. It also meant he would have to gnaw at his life savings, affecting his children's future education, his current rented stay and their whole lives.

At the advice of a distant relative, Manoj brought Saikrishna to our treatment unit, hoping for a miracle. As with every patient we encounter, this was a battle we were proud to fight for the patients on behalf of their families. But we are not gods or saints who can work miracles. As doctors, we were equipped with only these contrivances—the power of medical science and the optimism of evidence-based medicine to rationally utilize every possible armamentarium of diagnostic and therapeutic options against this young girl's worsening condition.

I looked at her clinical condition and recent blood reports. I knew this would likely end up in one of two ways: with her dying or with her having a successful, life-saving liver transplantation.

I admitted the deeply jaundiced girl with fluid in her abdomen and reviewed all her investigations with laser-precise attentiveness. The features of Wilson's disease were there, of this there was no doubt. However, so was autoimmune hepatitis, which was a rare possibility, but strange, given the current circumstances. How could two very different disease conditions work in tandem to injure the same organ? Saikrishna did not have a clearly identifiable or pre-existing liver disease and a predisposing risk factor for her current liver ailment. Two vastly different liver diseases—one autoimmune and the other genetic—co-existing in a young patient was unreal. She was just a little girl enjoying her life, school, friends and family.

I gazed at the records again. And again. Something was missing. There could have been a primary event creating confusion in the minds of all the doctors who had treated her before.

A distraction.

A red herring.

If so, then what was damaging her liver?

~

Medical science, and diagnosis, is a systematic process. It is not based on whims, fancies or blind assumptions. It is a methodical flow of confirmed and tested validations that takes a physician on a path that starts from an observation (or observations) and ends in the most attainable truth on outcomes under given circumstances. The methodical flow is algorithmic.

Algorithms lead the way on the path to diagnosis; clinical algorithms are a physician's strongest ally. And so, in this case of mine, we applied diagnostic algorithms for Wilson's disease first.

In April 2001, a large group of liver disease experts convened in Leipzig, Germany, to formulate what would come to be known as 'The Leipzig Criteria' for diagnosing Wilson's disease. A scoring system was created based on seven clinical and investigational variables, with a score of 4 or more considered a definitive diagnosis of Wilson's disease. In Saikrishna, a final score of 3 meant a Wilson's disease diagnosis was possible, but more tests were needed to confirm it.

The diagnosis of autoimmune hepatitis was far more challenging because it can mimic other liver conditions, and its symptoms and lab results can vary significantly from person to person. However, an early diagnosis was important because immunosuppression is life-saving. In 2008, clinical researchers from eleven centres worldwide gathered to simplify the diagnosis of autoimmune hepatitis. The outcome of that gathering was based on six clinical points and blood investigations—after which a score of more than 6 was probable diagnosis and above seven was a definite one. In Saikrishna's case, this score was 6, which meant we required an additional investigation in the form of a liver biopsy to confirm a definite diagnosis of autoimmune hepatitis. By now, Manoj had little money left, and genetic testing, which was the next step, was expensive.

Hippocrates once said, 'Where the art of medicine is loved, there is also love for humanity.' As doctors, we need to remember this the most.

I paid for the genetic testing from my salary, and the samples were sent to a specialized lab in Pune, Maharashtra. It was now time for the liver to speak and open its Pandora's box so we could see what was happening. However, a liver biopsy was not easy in Saikrishna's case. She had liver failure, her blood was thin and she was at high risk of bleeding. The fluid in her abdomen made it impossible to pass a needle across the skin to sample the liver tissue. If it was done the usual way, using a percutaneous (through the skin) approach, then the chances of her bleeding into the abdomen from the liver surface were very high. So we called the experts with a new liver-biopsy technique to keep her out of harm's way. The chief of our interventional radiology department was an expert at tackling difficult-to-intervene cases like Saikrishna.

In 1883, Dr Paul Ehrlich ventured into uncharted medical territory, piercing the skin with a large-bore needle to extract liver tissue. However, his efforts yielded samples too scant for meaningful study. Just before the Second World War, Danish physicians Iversen and Roholm refined the technique, harnessing the power of negative pressure to draw richer specimens, shedding light on the enigma of acute hepatitis. In 1940, the introduction of the Silverman needle revolutionized the procedure by producing well-formed cylindrical tissue cores, though bleeding risks remained. Seeking swiftness and precision, Giorgio Menghini later introduced a needle so deft it captured tissue in a heartbeat, cementing the foundation of modern liver biopsy. However, in cases of advanced liver failure, traditional methods posed significant bleeding risks, leading Charles Theodore Dotter to propose a novel approach in 1964: accessing the liver through a large neck vein. Three years later, doctors William Hanafee and Marvin Weiner transformed vision into reality, performing the first transjugular liver biopsy in humans—a triumph of science that forever altered the landscape of medicine.

Five decades after this new and safe method was first described, Saikrishna went in for a transjugular liver biopsy. Within minutes, a long needle and a wire went through her neck to reach her blood vessel within the liver, traversing her beating heart and prominent veins. This method could extract the liver tissue for our pathologist to see under the microscope for a final diagnosis. Everything was done without any risk of bleeding. The pathologist was notified that we needed results within forty-eight hours because a young girl's life was at stake. Saikrishna was getting sicker daily, and her abdominal fluid was increasing. While we waited for the biopsy reports, Saikrishna was put on diuretics and a salt-restricted diet to remove excess fluid in her abdomen through the urine.

Time was ticking away. Before the end of two days, I received a call from the pathology department.

'Ask the patient to stop drinking alcohol. The liver biopsy is highly suggestive of alcohol-related hepatitis,' my senior pathologist remarked from the other end.

'So much fat inside the liver cells, inflammation around fatty liver cells, and a pattern of liver injury and scarring that is very consistent with severe alcohol-related liver disease,' she went on.

If there were anything in the liver, I would trust my senior pathologist to identify it in the blink of an eye. Perplexed, I told her, 'But, ma'am, this is a fourteen-year-old girl. There is, without doubt, no history of consumption of alcohol or alcohol-use disorder.' She rechecked the patient's details to confirm that the biopsy was, indeed, that of fourteen-year-old Saikrishna. I could hear her mind working at the other end of the phone. 'There is something more,' she said. 'You see, the severe alcohol-related liver injury is masking something else.'

She told me, 'There is only one way to address this. You will have to treat and reverse the alcohol-related liver injury and subject the child to another liver biopsy. This will help us identify the second hit to her liver.' But for us to do that, Saikrishna had to survive.

I asked my pathologist, 'How is this possible? Alcohol-related injury on top of another unidentifiable liver disease. It is very bizarre.'

She responded calmly, 'You are missing something from clinical history. Keep her alive so that we can diagnose her.'

The father's words kept playing in my mind like a terrifying death loop: 'Liver transplantation is not an option.' A young girl child had alcohol-related hepatitis. We were not ready to embrace death. Not yet.

It was enough to make me lose my sleep.

Regeneration

The next day started early. I skipped coffee and sat down with Saikrishna's parents. In my outpatient office, I asked them, with police inquiry precision, everything about their daughter's diet and use of any alcohol-based drugs or supplements. Their reply to everything was a 'no', until the mother said, 'What about her anti-seizure syrups?'

I sat up and repeated, 'Anti-seizure?'

I was furious but kept myself in check.

'Why did you not tell me Saikrishna was on medicines for seizure control?'

The father replied, 'But, sir, these are not medications. These are natural supplements prescribed by our local Ayurvedic practitioner.'

My hearing sharpened as every little noise around me died down.

Saikrishna had suffered from childhood seizures in November 2013. She was started on the anti-seizure drug phenytoin, which she took for three months. Unfortunately, she developed seizures while she was on medication, after which additional anti-seizure drugs were advised. The family had then decided to consult an Ayurvedic practitioner near their home for 'safer and natural' alternative medicines for seizure control.

From May 2014 onwards, she had taken the Ayurvedic medications, prescribed from a local and well-known centre for seizure control.

Astonished, I asked the parents to bring and show me the Ayurvedic medications. The child was on nine different kinds of traditional and proprietary herbal medications. Interestingly, these included *arishtams*, Ayurvedic medicines prepared by boiling medicinal herbs in water and fermenting the decoction. These decoctions usually contain herbs such as the fire flame bush (*Woodfordia fruticose*) or dhataki, as it is commonly known. When boiled in water along with added sugar, herbs such as this generate alcohol during fermentation. There were also *asavams*, a type of Ayurvedic medicine prepared by the fermentation of fresh herbal juices, also containing self-generated alcohol; and *churna*s, a mixture of powdered herbs and metal and mineral preparations, in addition to a wide variety of coloured pills and capsules with unlabelled multi-herbal ingredients.

'How much was she on, and for how long?' I asked her father.

'Sir, it has been going on for three years, and we have lost count of the bottles we have bought. We never stopped these herbal medicines and supplements as she has never had a seizure episode since starting them,' he told me, a bit disconcerted by my questioning, I could see.

Arishtams and asavams are used for various disease conditions and are supposed to have medicinal value. Nonetheless, the evidence for such therapeutic benefits only exists within ancient Ayurvedic textual references and in the testimonials of people's personal experiences. There are none proven with objective evidence or validation from a scientific standpoint.

The presence of alcohol in arishtams is well known, so much so that during a statewide restriction on alcohol use by the government, people flocked to Ayurvedic shops to buy and get high on the 'medicinal' herbal drink. Ayurvedic 'alcoholic' medications saw increased sales during the Covid-related lockdown. Arishtam and asavam contain anywhere between 10 per cent (in classical preparations) and 30 per cent (in poor-quality manufactured decoctions) ethanol (or ethyl alcohol)—the type of alcohol in standard beverages such as beer, wine and hard liquors.

Saikrishna was on multiple alcohol-based herbal formulations for her seizure disorder for over three years. However, despite my suspicions, I wanted to confirm that the source of alcohol that resulted in this young girl's severe alcohol-associated hepatitis was from the Ayurvedic medicinal supplements. So we retrieved the liquid herbal formulations, sent them out for chemical and toxicology analyses, for which we again paid from our pockets to reduce the burden on Manoj. I knew he was running from pillar to post, begging and borrowing funds to clear his daughter's hospital bills.

Meanwhile, the genetic testing reports from Pune arrived and were negative for mutations associated with Wilson's disease. Everyone heaved a sigh of relief. But we had much work to be done. Since alcohol-associated hepatitis was confirmed on her liver biopsy, we now had some clues to start potentially beneficial treatment. But the question loomed: How do we decide what the best treatment option was for her?

In the late 1950s, European clinicians began exploring the use of steroids to treat alcohol-related cirrhosis, seeking a remedy for the devastating effects of liver disease. Among them, John Joseph Webster pioneered the administration of adrenal gland extracts, harnessing the power of hormonal corticosteroids to combat cirrhosis and its complications, bringing relief through reduced inflammation, improved appetite and a renewed sense of well-being. Decades later, in 1978, Professor Willis C. Maddrey at Johns Hopkins Hospital led a groundbreaking clinical trial, demonstrating that prednisolone therapy significantly lowered early mortality in patients suffering from severe alcohol-associated hepatitis. Despite countless studies on alternative treatments, steroids remained the only intervention proven to offer short-term survival—an enduring testament to their efficacy, even as fate cruelly forced young Saikrishna, a teetotaller, into this very diagnosis, leaving no choice but to initiate steroid therapy without delay.

While we waited for Saikrishna's response to the steroid therapy, we got an email from the toxicology lab that tested the young girl's herbal decoctions. Two out of four liquid formulations tested positive for alcohol. Worryingly, the cumulative alcohol content was 26 per cent volume by volume levels, far more than in beer and wine. The three years that Saikrishna had taken these *supposed* anti-seizure medicines had ensured they slowly gnawed at her liver, until she developed alcohol-associated hepatitis.

When I prescribed steroids for the little girl, my hands froze and then trembled while I wrote orders for prednisolone. It is easy to prescribe, but at times it is challenging to cope with the consequences of that prescription, especially when you know that what you prescribe is a double-edged sword. In the studies on severe alcohol-associated hepatitis, steroid therapy was associated with adverse outcomes in some. Patients developed severe infections or died of bleeding as an adverse event. Even though this was notable in a small number, most patients experienced the benefits of steroid therapy.

Nonetheless, the steroids were doing what they were supposed to do. Without fail, Saikrishna's total bilirubin levels dropped every week, starting at 26 mg/dL from the start of therapy to 4.2 mg/dL at the end of four weeks.

I had not expected this. I kept playing the death of this young girl in my mind and comforting myself that I was doing the best that could be done. The sigh of relief every week when the jaundice levels went down awakened the same excitement in her parents and me. But I always kept a confident and stiff face, signalling the child's parents that everything was going according to my plan. It was not. I did not know whose plan it was that we were all playing out, but all I had was the comfort that the work of scientists, researchers and clinicians—that of the evidence-based medicine that came before me—provided a path to walk on, showing me a way forward.

But there was still one question that lurked at the back of my mind: What if Saikrishna were to, unfortunately, develop complications due to steroids? What if she died of an infection? What if she developed a bleed and became moribund? Wouldn't that be my doing? That I took a patient many steps forward and then abandoned her because I made a choice that was not foolproof?

Sir William Osler, the Canadian physician and the father of bedside medical training, once said, 'Medicine is a science of uncertainty and an art of probability.' Embracing uncertainty in clinical medicine makes a doctor more humane. Doubting one's decision opens vulnerabilities that require a physician to think outside the box and learn new things about tackling that knowledge gap. A self-questioning physician is far better than one who hides behind a made-up wall of confidence.

After her steroid course was complete, Saikrishna was free from jaundice. She did not develop infections or bleeding. Her appetite returned, she felt better and wanted to return to school. But we had only won the battle and were ready for war. Saikrishna's *real* war. It was time for us to look at the liver again. We had kept her alive to diagnose the underlying liver condition for real.

I told Manoj that a second biopsy was required. And without thinking twice, in the blink of an eye, he said, 'Sir, she has come this far, and we know how your team has been working hard. You look exhausted. But you keep going at it.'

I was exhausted. I wanted this to end—but I wanted this to end with Saikrishna going home. I was tired because I had not slept well in weeks, thinking about how this girl could be sent home hale and hearty.

Manoj continued, 'My daughter is now under your care. This place is a hospital. Here, people come for treatment—some walk in and never go back, and some come unconscious but walk back home. This place is brooding, but your presence here makes it my sanctuary. Please take care of her and give her back to me when you know she is safe.'

My responsibilities now felt like mountains placed on my shoulders, and this stress was reflected in my sleep. I had become an insomniac.

A second biopsy was done. This time, we could go across the skin between Saikrishna's lower ribs because her liver functions had improved, her blood was not thin anymore and the fluid in her abdomen had disappeared. A plain old routine liver biopsy.

A strong girl. What a fighter!

At the brink of liver failure, a liver transplant candidate was looking Death right in the eyes. Moreover, two liver biopsies. Most adults cringe at the mention of the word 'biopsy' because among laypersons it has always been associated with the dreaded 'C word': cancer. The fact is, a biopsy, especially one of the liver, is not only to diagnose cancer but also to understand the cause of a liver condition, the severity of the disease and to help doctors identify patterns of liver damage that could help them realize the best treatment options for the patient. Some patterns of liver damage would result in early death and require decisions for an early liver transplant.

If this little girl could go through with this, I had to go with her.

After the second biopsy, Saikrishna was discharged from daycare after a brief period of observation. In the meantime, she continued the low-dose medicines to control the swelling in the abdomen and legs, and the addition of a group of drugs called beta-blockers that help reduce increased liver pressures associated with severe liver disease and help prevent bleeding from blood vessels in the food pipe and stomach.

Four days later, while I was seeing a new patient in my outpatient office, the senior pathologist called me, asking me to join her in her office. I rushed to her and looked at the images of the little girl's pieces of liver in hues of pink and blue projected on the computer screen. Saikrishna's second biopsy was unlike anything we had expected.

'Have you heard of a condition called hepato-portal sclerosis?' she asked me.

I nodded.

I had read about it in my medical textbooks and written short and long essays about it for my theory exams.

Had I seen it in real life?

Never.

Not until now.

To understand the mysterious disease entity called hepato-portal sclerosis, one must understand the normal liver and the cirrhotic liver. In a normal liver, under the microscope, the liver cells (also called hepatocytes) are arranged in a beautiful sun ray pattern around blood vessels. In a cirrhotic liver, due to long-term insult from a damaging cause, such as alcohol or a chronic viral infection, the beautiful pattern is lost.

Instead, the liver cells become clustered into nodules surrounded by scar tissue—also known as fibrosis. The nodular arrangement of liver cells, encircled by thick, fibrous scars, gives the cirrhotic liver its distinct irregular and shrunken appearance. This leads to another significant event inside the cirrhotic liver. The shrinkage, nodules and scars increase pressure inside the main vessel, supplying blood into the liver, called the portal vein. This increase in pressure within the liver is called 'portal hypertension', which is the sole reason cirrhosis patients bleed and develop fluid build-up in the abdomen (called ascites) and chest (called hydrothorax)—as Saikrishna did. Also associated with portal hypertension was an enlarged spleen, mainly because the high pressures in the portal vein get transmitted back to the spleen through its vein connections. However, there was a group of diseases in which liver pressures went high without cirrhosis, leading to bleeds and abdominal fluid collection. This was called non-cirrhotic portal hypertension, or portal hypertension in the absence of cirrhosis.

Hepato-portal sclerosis was a peculiar form of non-cirrhotic portal hypertension. Almost 250 years ago, Dr F.L. Bang described a patient with complications of portal hypertension presenting with abdominal fluid and bleeding without cirrhosis. Decade after decade, similar cases were being reported. But intriguingly, all these patients had something else in common—they suffered from a skin condition called psoriasis. They were on a peculiar treatment with an externally applied medicine called Fowler's Solution. The others who did not use Fowler's Solution did ingest the main ingredient in the solution through other sources.

In 1999, clinical scientists from the department of medicine and gastroenterology at the Institute of Postgraduate Medical Education and Research, Calcutta (now Kolkata), described more than 200 patients with non-cirrhotic portal hypertension in whom the common agent implicated came from a groundwater source that the affected persons used to consume daily.

This was not all.

In 1786, Thomas Fowler published the use of a particular medicine to cure fevers and intermittent headaches. Later, it was used broadly to treat cancers and skin diseases such as psoriasis. Patients using Fowler's Solution on a long-term basis developed various well-characterized clinical features apart from liver disease and associated portal hypertension: skin pigmentation and neurological disorders, such as tremors, poor concentration and peripheral nerve inflammation and damage.

When I looked at the liver-biopsy pictures, they had everything described decades ago in patients using Fowler's Solution. The liver damage was peculiar—only minimal inflammation now because all the significant inflammation seen previously due to alcohol-associated hepatitis had settled. There was no necrosis (loss of liver cells) or nodule formation. But scarring was present, and its pattern was unlike what we see in cirrhosis. The area of the liver where the major blood vessels and bile duct traverse through, called the portal region, was deeply scarred, the condition now known as hepato-portal sclerosis.

But what was causing it?

I leaned back on the chair and closed my eyes. I surrounded myself with silence and took significant steps back to look at Saikrishna's whole clinical picture again, back to the beginning. The young girl had pigmentation across her upper arms and body, tremors, poor concentration and high liver pressures with fluid in the abdomen, but no cirrhosis.

And then, I looked at my pathologist and she looked at me.

I thanked her because she had unlocked the final piece in this puzzle, and all I had to do was confirm it.

I knew the cause of Saikrishna's liver disease was dangling right in front of my eyes, but I sincerely hoped I was wrong, for if I was right, Saikrishna's war against a terrible foe had only just begun.

~

The reason for portal hypertension and the peculiar liver disease in those who consumed Fowler's Solution and those who ingested contaminated groundwater was the presence of the inorganic heavy metal arsenic, a potent systemic toxin. Fowler's Solution contains 1 per cent potassium arsenate, and the inorganic arsenic in contaminated water sources poses a considerable risk for chronic toxicity, primarily affecting the liver, brain, nerves and skin.

There was only one thing to do—I had to confront Saikrishna's father again.

'There were other Ayurvedic medicines, too, right?' I asked Manoj.

'Yes,' he told me. 'Powders and pills too.'

'Retrieve them for me, please. I want to confirm something, and then we end this terrible ordeal. Also, I would like to have hair and nail samples from you, your wife, Saikrishna and her sibling too.'

'Why?' he asked me worryingly. 'Is it for more analysis? Will it cost us this time?'

I looked at him and assured him that the costs would be resolved. To be honest, at this stage I had little more to spare for the tests from my month's salary, which meant ordering less food and restricting shopping over the weekends with my family.

Nine more traditional Ayurvedic supplements were retrieved and sent for analysis.

In a better world, arsenic should not be detected in drugs, medicines and health supplements. But here we were with the results revealing detectable arsenic in six out of nine samples analysed, ranging from 44.3 to 1982 mg/kg, which was, at maximum, 1,00,000 times more than the limit recommended for drinking water. Saikrishna was unintentionally being poisoned with arsenic under the garb of natural and safe herbal medicines. But we had to be sure. Arsenic was found in the herbal medication. But was the young girl getting poisoned with it?

In 2008, a team of doctors from the department of dermatology and venereology, All India Institute of Medical Sciences (AIIMS), New Delhi, had identified an eleven-year-old girl, just like Saikrishna, who developed severe skin manifestations and liver disease due to arsenic poisoning. The girl had seizures and was on multiple Ayurvedic formulations for six to eighteen months. An analysis of eight Ayurvedic supplements retrieved from the parents and the young girl's blood had revealed high arsenic levels.

And I wondered.

How many more Saikrishnas were out there who would be going through the same avoidable health burden right now, and would not have to face a life-or-death situation if they knew about this and threw away their untested herbal supplements right at this moment?

Arsenic has a peculiar feature—it has a high affinity for a particular amino acid called cysteine that makes up proteins in the body. Cysteine is abundant in the protein called keratin, which makes up hair and nails. Detection of arsenic above a certain threshold in hair and nails is confirmation of chronic arsenic poisoning. Saikrishna's hair and nails showed very high levels of arsenic, but not her parents' or sibling's—which only meant one thing.

There was no common source, and only the girl was exposed to it, which eliminated water as the source of arsenic. As all the shattered pieces of this complex puzzle fell into place, I was getting breathless. Saikrishna was constantly and consistently being poisoned with arsenic, without her knowing it, and the source of that arsenic was the supposed herbal medicines prescribed to protect her from seizures.

After a roller-coaster ride of medical investigations, we finally had a diagnosis: severe alcohol-associated hepatitis due to Ayurvedic decoctions and non-cirrhotic portal hypertension due to chronic arsenic poisoning from Ayurvedic herbal supplements. Even though the girl escaped the disastrous alcohol liver injury, the scars from arsenic on her body were here to stay.

The liver is a marvellous organ. In stress, it tries to grow. In injury, it heals itself. When under pressure, it grows to overcome. Once we knew what was stressing Saikrishna's liver, we gave it a chance to rebuild, reconstruct and regenerate. After six months of aggressive evaluation, complex investigations and targeted therapies, young Saikrishna was allowed to go home but had to revisit for more extended follow-up investigations and cancer surveillance.

Before they left, I met her father, Manoj.

He came close and told me, 'I can go home because you kept your promise. I can now spend time with my daughter, and this time gained is like a bonus for me. I do not care what the future holds.'

The future was bleak. But I did not tell him that. Not yet. Chronic arsenic poisoning brings out its ugly head in the long term. The biggest challenge to preserving life came with the development of skin cancer, a type of liver and kidney cancer called angiosarcoma, and urinary bladder and lung cancers. Saikrishna would be on surveillance for these monsters all her life.

Her journey would be mine and mine, hers.

I had a recurring dream that she outlived me in this life.

Before we said our goodbyes, Manoj told me, 'It is strange. Such poisons as medicines, but Krishna never had problems with her seizures again.'

Then I let the last piece in the puzzle fall into place.

Saikrishna never had seizures while on the multiple herbal drugs because they were adulterated with a modern medicine called clonazepam, a well-known anti-seizure drug. It was not because of the herbal pills.

Our analysis had picked that up too.

Heaving a sigh and staying silent, probably deep in thought about his folly, Manoj bade me farewell until our next follow-up meeting.

~

It has been nine years now.

The girl is well and acing her studies. Her tremors are gone. Her memory is sharp. She has her good and bad days like any normal child. But the chronic liver disease and arsenic did something to her body. Her menstrual cycles were erratic and she was referred to a gynaecologist for hormonal treatment. The dark cloud of cancer looming above her future and the possibility that she may become infertile would not bring her the simple joys in life.

I sit through these thoughts almost every day.

I am hoping against all odds that the day will never come when I have to see her again and diagnose her with a heart-wrenching event due to the arsenic that is slowly eating her from inside because herbal medicines were considered natural and safe for a child to have.

An avoidable health burden.

I worry whenever Saikrishna has her follow-up health check with me. After my outpatient work finishes, before I leave for home, I look through the next day's appointments and see if her name is on the list. If it is there, the rest of the day comes crashing down on me.

I sit on the chair at night, watching my little daughters, Alanna and Aideen, sleep. I look at them and see how quickly and peacefully they move into a deep sleep. I put off the main lights but keep the warm purple fairy lights on. I step out silently to my room, where my wife, Teena, and my littlest son, Arthur, are fast asleep. I quietly slide under the covers and place my phone on the bedside table. My eyes remain open, and I stare at the warm, yellow-lit ceiling.

I try to sleep, but I see Saikrishna's face and think about her parents. Her little brother.

Their simple lives.

Their unforeseen future.

I see her father's dreary face again and again.

Hepatology is the study of liver disease and the art of preserving liver health. I may be biased here, but it is the most extreme form of internal medicine. From head to toe, a liver doctor's knowledge about the human body must be sharp and clear. The liver holds all organs in an embrace. When attacked, it is bittersweet how the liver tries hard, until overwhelmed, to preserve everything through selfless regeneration. It is a forgiving organ.

The study and practice of preserving the liver, which unconditionally tries to maintain us, is depressing and exhilarating. It wears me out but also pumps me full of life. It satisfies me with regretful pleasantness.

I am in this now. Knee-deep.

I am not going to wade out of this pool. I am going to swim against the currents.

I am not alone. I have patients I hold on to. Families that hold on to us both. We are all in this together.

But I am tired, and my eyes feel heavy, and I hear it in whispers.

I hear it again. I know I will keep hearing it.

Every moment of my waking. Every time that I try to sleep.

Every day is a battle. Every case, a war.

These are our stories of love, loss and regeneration.

I hear it again as my eyes shut heavy, and finally, the slumber takes over me.

She has been advised to undergo a liver transplant to prolong her life. We are poor. Can you please help us avoid it?

I yield to my lassitude with a weary smile.

I have seized the day.

I am not breathless anymore.

Tomorrow is another day.

The words of Rumi echo through my mind: 'I know you are tired, but come, this is the way.'

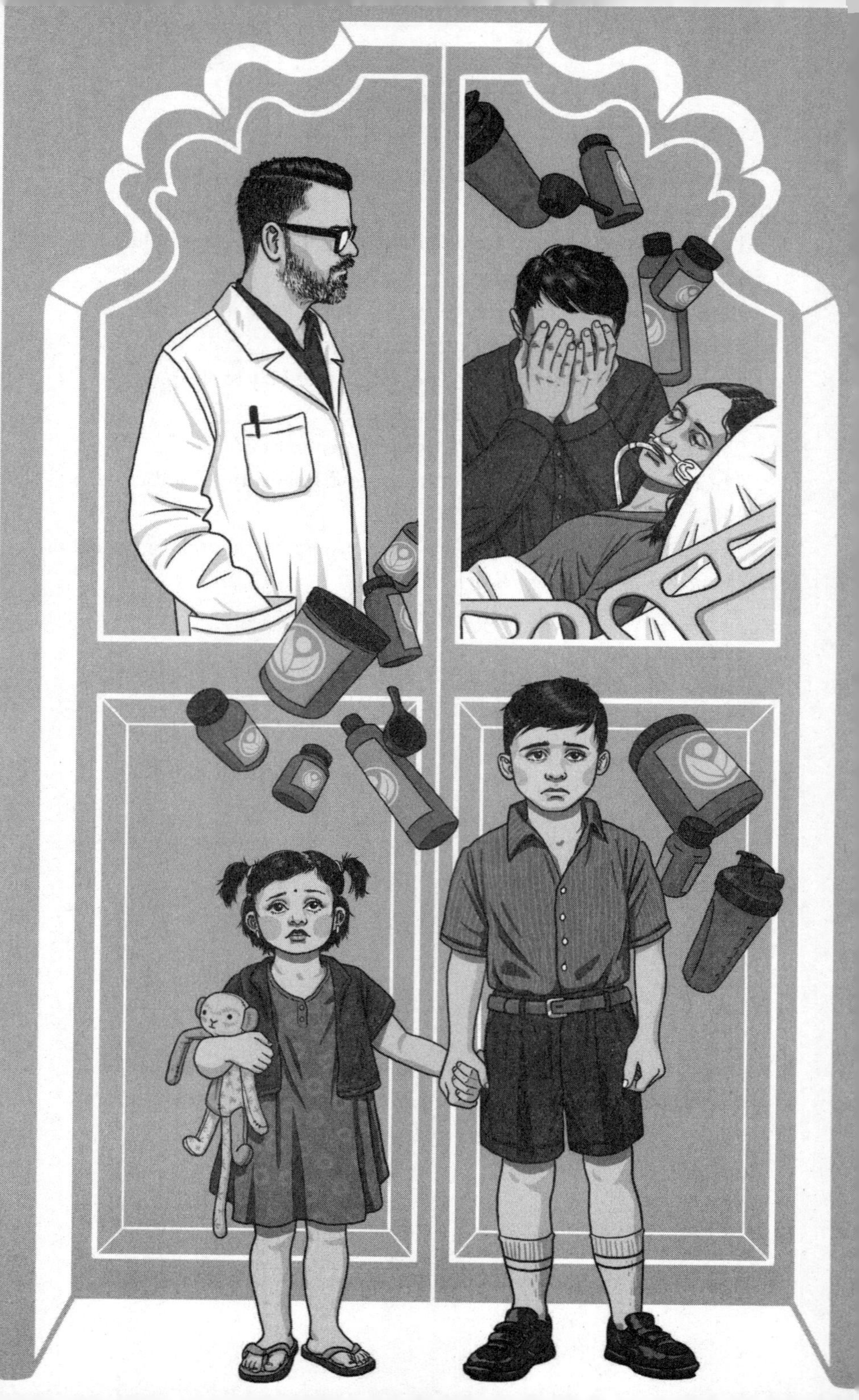

CHAPTER 1

The Titan God of Fire

Understanding Liver Failure and Regeneration

The Nightmare Circus

'Family means nobody gets left behind, or forgotten.'
—DAVID OGDEN STIERS

A Port in the Storm

MY ELDEST DAUGHTER WAS BORN ON A MILDLY HUMID, warm evening in November 2013 in Thiruvananthapuram (formerly Trivandrum) in Kerala. I was in New Delhi, training for my hepatology speciality at the Institute of Liver and Biliary Sciences. My wife gave birth surrounded by strangers in blue and green scrubs inside a secluded room. I think about that day whenever I am lost in thought on a break on a routine weekday.

There are some things that I—we—take for granted. But looking back, even though I regret some decisions, they were unavoidable, nonetheless. Hepatology residency and training were heartbreaking and mind-numbing. Medical studies in India are exhausting; you enter a human but come out a humanoid. Lost for feeling and hardened to emotions. You see so much death that death becomes part of life.

Sometimes I feel that studying medicine changed me in unexpected ways. I miss the boy that I was. I miss growing up.

When I was that boy returning home from school, I remember the perfectly elevated wall that surrounded our rented home back at the quaint little village called Chungam, in the quiet suburb of Kottayam town. The wall overlooked a small rice field surrounded by water and was just good enough for me to lean on. Sometimes I would put in a fishing line and catch a catfish, sometimes a turtle would attack my line. Even when I did not catch anything, I was still content with that view, that place, that moment frozen in time. This memory became my sanctuary.

I had been through my bachelor's and master's degrees in medical training for more than a decade before my hepatology residency, and somehow, somewhere—and I cannot figure this out even now—I lost touch with my human self but grew one for others in the process. The small rice field, the brick wall at the perfect height and the lake that contained surprises were replaced by desks, soiled beds, blood on the floor, urine bags, breathing tubes and sweat and tears—surrounded by four walls that absorbed all the wailing, even the silent kind. This was what years of medical training and practice of medicine did to me, and I am sure to many others.

Sometimes when I felt overwhelmingly sad by the death of a child—because everyone is someone's child—I would let myself cry under the fully open shower inside the bathroom. It was my own satisfying way to cope. Outside that deafening shower, I was still the confident doctor in a white coat, ready to take on the world of illness and misery. My profession became my life, and life became a formality. Never a day off after a thirty-six-hour shift, learning to work by skipping meals, and staying sharp and clear in thoughts and decision-making even after compromising on precious sleep hours were additional lessons learnt apart from the practice of medicine.

In this process, doctors get lost. Lost for words, lost for actions, lost in thoughts about chances and opportunities that are small but matter significantly in retrospect. Like the birth of my eldest daughter. We named her Alanna, from the Old High German word for 'precious' or the Irish term 'a leanbh' for 'child'. Before I left for Thiruvananthapuram in a hurry, catching the last flight out of New Delhi, I looked at the cutest little plush bunny from outside a shop window.

The next thing I knew, the bunny was inside my travel bag on the way to Thiruvananthapuram. It was for my wife, Teena. I remember these little things even now. I do not know when I landed, or when or how I got to the hospital room to embrace Teena or hold my child for the first time. But I remember the embrace, and I still feel the warmth of that hold. Looking back, I regret that similar, more intoxicating memories could not have been made. This was life. Every day was special. We were a family, and I had never felt this way. This was a special moment, and family was forever.

When patients are entrusted to my care, my primal response is to ask them about their families. Do they have any? Do they live together? How close are they? Do they have only each other? Are they in this fight together but feel lonely? Without letting them know, I willingly and gladly join them in their chaos because family is everything.

~

On a humid and warm morning in November 2017, such chaos was imminent. I received an unexpected call from the emergency department.

'There is a self-referred patient for you,' the emergency doctor on call told me.

'Self-referred?' I asked him.

'Yes,' he confirmed, 'the husband has previously got his sick wife discharged from multiple hospitals looking for a diagnosis. Says this place is his last hope.'

Self-referrals were always ominous. It meant that doctors were lost, the patient was extremely sick and, most importantly, the family was on the verge of a breakdown. As I walked into the emergency room, I found myself looking at a profoundly jaundiced, disoriented woman lying on the trolley bed.

Her husband, with his folded hands, was beckoning me for help.

I obliged.

Unknown to me at the time, my acceptance of that patient would eventually tear me apart and drive my treating unit into disarray.

But from the corner of my eye, I saw something else.

I saw them. The two children, a girl and a boy, at the leg-end of the gurney, watching their mother go in and out of a coma.

If a family is an island holding against a storm, a mother is the port in the storm. An asylum, a sanctuary that held everything together.

I looked at the children. It seemed as if they were about to lose that sanctuary, and I was the only one standing in between, hopelessly.

The moment I saw the patient, I knew she was battling one of the most terrifying diseases in medical practice—a condition called acute liver failure or ALF. We needed a cause for the liver failure, and we needed it fast.

A Forgiving Organ

Raj worked at a small clinic as a physician's help. His wife, Meera, was thirty-two years old. They had an elder daughter and a younger son. About seven weeks prior to their hospital visit, Meera had started losing her appetite. Seeing meat dishes on the table made her nauseous. Every day was a chore. She would get up early, prepare lunch for the children and make breakfast for Raj before he left for the clinic. This continued for a few days until she could not get up from the bed one day. A concerned Raj called in an emergency leave and took Meera to a nearby clinic. The doctors prescribed her multivitamins and asked them to return within a week if things did not settle. They said it was 'the flu'. A couple of days later, Meera started feeling worse and, for the first time, noticed that her urine was a deep yellow. Raj found that the whites of her eyes were also tinged with yellow.

Meera had jaundice. Being in the medical field for a while, Raj knew this was not the flu, and rushed Meera to the emergency centre of the nearest big hospital. Seeing how lethargic she was, the doctors advised admission for further evaluation. The initial blood reports showed that the liver values were inflated. Meera's total bilirubin (the blood test for jaundice) was 11 (normal is less than 1 mg/dl) and her liver enzymes—aspartate transaminase (also called AST or SGOT) and alanine transaminase (ALT or SGPT)—were in the thousands (normal is approximately less than 40–50 U/L). An increase in these enzymes suggested hepatitis (or liver inflammation). AST is also present in the heart, the skeletal muscles and the red blood cells. This makes ALT more indicative of liver cell damage than AST. In Meera's case, the ALT elevation was much higher than AST, making the source of her jaundice and her illness directly related to ongoing liver disease.

An ultrasound scan revealed that Meera's liver was enlarged and swollen, but there was nothing to suggest that she had pre-existing liver disease. The doctors were sure this was a case of acute hepatitis with jaundice. Since jaundice is not a disease but a symptom or sign of a larger disease, the next best practice was to identify the cause. A panel of tests were ordered, and while patiently waiting for the results, Meera was put on a protein-rich diet—to be consumed in small, frequent meals—along with medication, to reduce nausea and improve appetite.

Contrary to traditional beliefs, restricting food intake during acute liver disease worsens a patient's clinical status. The liver does not 'need to rest' when there is jaundice. In ancient Greece, physician philosophers treated patients with acute jaundice in various ways. Seeing a yellow bird and bloodletting from the right arm were both believed to be cures. Dietary restrictions included fish and milk, and strong laxatives were used to cleanse the bowel of 'toxins' and 'evils'.

Meera was holding on even though her lethargy worsened and the fatigue became crippling. To everyone's surprise, the initial blood work revealed no contributory findings towards a diagnosis. Tests for common viral infections that could have contributed to hepatitis were also negative. Autoimmune hepatitis, a disease explained in brief in the prologue, predominantly seen in women, was also ruled out on the basis of blood tests. Meera was not on any prolonged medications except for thyroid hormone supplementation for hypothyroidism. There was no recent history of antibiotics or painkillers being taken that could injure the liver.

The doctors were stumped. But they did not expect what was coming next. Five days after her admission, Meera's liver values started to skyrocket and her blood started losing its power to clot—a condition called 'coagulation failure', which happens with progressive severe liver injury. This was noted on a test called the prothrombin time and international normalized ratio (PT/INR, in short). The liver makes the proteins that help the blood coagulate (to maintain viscosity or thickness) during an injury to arrest bleeding, and helps maintain a balance in the blood between pro-coagulants (which make the blood thicker) and anticoagulants (which make the blood thinner). The normal range for PT is 10 to 13 seconds, and INR is 1.1 or below.

Coagulation failure is diagnosed when the PT exceeds test control by six seconds and the INR goes above 1.5. Meera's INR was now 2.1, which meant her liver injury was severe and failure of the organ was impending. To make matters worse, the hospital did not have a dedicated team to care for critically ill liver-disease patients, and so, taking the high path and acknowledging their deficiencies, the doctors advised referral to a higher centre.

Late that evening Raj took Meera to a hospital well known for treating advanced liver-disease patients, with his children by Meera's side; his mother came along for additional support. Meera was admitted to the medical ICU through an emergency referral service for upgraded management. Raj, his children and his mother waited outside until a room was prepared for them.

ICU specialists closely reviewed Meera's blood tests and clinical notes from the previous hospital and were sure that Meera would end up with ALF.

Raj began running helter-skelter for funds to continue Meera's treatment. But the doctors were clear that all the money being spent now would only be for supportive care and that a new liver was the only way for Meera to survive. Moreover, it would cost massive amounts of money for post-transplant medical management.

Even at this juncture, however, doctors could not figure out the cause of Meera's severe hepatitis. They did everything they could to keep the liver going, but saw that their efforts were eclipsed by the unforgiving condition eating away at Meera's liver.

~

Among the organs of the human body, the liver has the most extraordinary regenerative capacity. Even after toxins, drugs and alcohol, it bounces back to stabilize its volume, mass and functions. The liver is forgiving, but like everything else, it has a limit and can be overwhelmed, which then leads to ALF.

Humanity's initial curiosity about liver regeneration was mainly founded on ancient mythology, on tales of supernatural vitality rather than on medical knowledge of the liver's regenerative abilities. Greek mythology talks about the punishment meted out to Prometheus, a Titan and the god of fire, by Zeus, the chief deity of the pantheon and the god of the sky and lightning. It is said that after the creation of humankind, while the mortals and immortals were feasting, Prometheus tricked Zeus into giving the best parts of the meal (the meat of slaughtered cows) to humans, and only fat and bones to the gods. Angered, Zeus revoked humankind's access to fire. But Prometheus stole the fire and returned it to humans, angering Zeus further. A raging Zeus ordered Hephaestus, the divine smith and the patron of craftsmen, to seize Prometheus and chain him to a rock on Mount Caucasus. Every morning, Zeus would send the Aetos Kaukasios, or the Caucasian Eagle, to feast on Prometheus's liver, only for it to grow back the next day and the ordeal to start all over again. This eternal punishment lasted for thirteen generations, until Hercules killed the eagle with his arrows. This was not the only documentation of liver regeneration in ancient mythology. The giant Tityus was banished to the underworld by Zeus for the rape and attack on Leto, the mother of Artemis and Apollo. There, two vultures feasted on his liver every new moon, which grew back every time, perpetuating the torture for eternity.

The interplay among liver injury, liver failure and liver regeneration is a complex process, and to confess, a mystery that medical science needs more time to understand fully. The liver has excellent resilience and can restore up to 70 per cent of its lost mass and function in just a few weeks. To study this process, surgeon researchers focused on the least appreciated animal from the human point of view—the rat.

In 1931, surgeons G.M. Higgins and R.M. Anderson removed 70 per cent of a white rat's liver and found that the leftover liver segments grew to increase and constitute approximately 45–70 per cent of the liver's original weight about twenty-four to seventy-two hours after the surgery. This was known as the partial hepatectomy (liver resection) model, or the PH model, which sparked further studies that paved the way for our current understanding of how the liver regenerates when under stress and loss.

The average lifespan of an adult liver cell varies from six to nine months. But when the liver is damaged, the cells suddenly become 'more alive' and kick into overdrive, re-enter the cell cycle and start dividing to produce more liver cells.

After a week of the surgery on the white rat, the weight of the liver increased by 5 per cent and at the end of two weeks it reached its original weight before surgery. This regeneration was the result of increased liver cell numbers (hyperplasia) and cell size (hypertrophy).

But there was something strange. When 30 per cent or less of the rodent's liver was removed, the regeneration did not kick in or, if it did, it started very slowly, primarily because of an increase in cell size and not the number. Additionally, when almost 90 per cent of the liver was removed, regeneration failed and the animal died.

The concept that only a tiny part of the liver was required for regeneration was known since ancient times. The Babylonian Talmud, the central text of Rabbinic Judaism and the primary source of Jewish religious law and theology, composed in 200–500 CE, states that the liver can successfully regenerate itself in humans even if only a part as small as an olive remains. But where was the liver getting the signal to start the regeneration process and why did this happen only under stress?

In 1951, Dr Nancy Bucher of the Massachusetts General Hospital in Boston, US, did something very intriguing. Her team used parabiotic rats for an experiment. Parabiosis is the surgical joining of two living organisms so they share a single physiological system. In this case, the two rats were made to share the same blood flowing through their systems so that when something was done to one rat, its consequences could be studied in the other. Dr Bucher's team removed two-thirds of the liver from one rat and found that the non-operated rat's liver showed signs of growth and cell division, thus proving that the signals for regeneration originated from the damaged liver. Through the secretion of enzymes and proteins, a complex network of signalling pathways originate from the damaged part of the liver to regulate the genes in the undamaged part to help recover lost liver mass.

There is a master gene signal that controls all of this. When the liver is damaged, the epithelial splicing regulator protein 2, or the ESRP2, drastically reduces in the viable liver cells. This protein is unique because its low levels transform the liver environment to that noted in a human foetus, and the rest of the liver is tricked into repopulating damaged areas through cell division and cell growth. The master gene signal pathway in the cells that ensured this is called the Hippo Pathway (short for the Salvador–Warts–Hippo Pathway), first described and studied in the fruit fly *Drosophila*, which was found to control tissue growth and organ size in animals—and for us, 'the hepatostat'. Much like a thermostat at home for controlling heating and cooling during seasons, a hepatostat, run by various complex signalling pathways in the liver, tells when the regeneration process needs to start and stop once the recovery of the lost liver tissue is complete. But when injury or stress to the liver is overwhelming, these signals fail, leading to liver failure.

This malfunction was already in motion in Meera's liver, as the organ function progressively deteriorated, demonstrated by rapidly rising jaundice and failing coagulation levels.

A Candle in the Wind

There are four prerequisites for a patient to be diagnosed with ALF: the liver must be healthy before the injury; there should be associated jaundice; evidence of blood thinning or coagulation failure reflected by the high INR test; and most importantly, a complication known as hepatic encephalopathy or, simply, brain failure. Meera had three of four, as her brain functions were intact—until the fourth day of admission to the ICU of the second hospital. Late one evening, the attending staff noticed that Meera was lost in thought. She was lying still on the bed, staring at the ceiling. When the staff member called out her name, she did not respond; instead, she asked the nurse where she was.

'You are in the hospital,' the kind nurse assured her.

'But it is time for school, and the children will be late,' Meera responded.

As an ICU nurse, she knew this was a bad sign. A terrible sign.

She rushed and called the duty doctor for a reassessment. When the doctor arrived, Meera was already mumbling. She needed clarification about the questions asked and was visibly confused in her responses.

'Please call her husband to the ICU,' the doctor told the staff without hesitation.

Brain dysfunction in liver disease, or hepatic encephalopathy, was the harbinger of death, bringing the diagnosis of ALF full circle. It meant two things. One, the liver had failed and could not handle the toxins and metabolic waste generated in the body. This toxic build-up in the blood, specifically ammonia, was bathing Meera's brain and causing its nerve cells and connections to misfire. Secondly, the exceptionally high level of ammonia in ALF leads to the swelling of brain cells: a condition called cerebral edema. This condition can rapidly progress to shut down brain functions, as the massively swollen brain—when it cannot expand further inside the skull—falls through natural holes within the skull bones (most commonly through the one situated at the back of the skull), killing the patient instantly due to a condition called 'brain herniation'. The only way to prevent this is an emergency liver transplant.

Clinically, the brain dysfunction in ALF progresses through various stages, starting from a mild lack of awareness in Stage I to a full-fledged coma in Stage IV. Meera was in Stage III, confused and on the brink of slipping into a coma, possibly to never return.

William Saunders described an ongoing 'sympathy' between the brain and the liver 220 years ago. In maniacal persons, this was disrupted when there was a defect in bile secretion. This was probably the first clear description of the relationship between the brain and liver axis in liver disease.

Hepatic encephalopathy and liver coma as a clinical entity came into light with the publication of separate case reports from 1833 to 1836 by doctors William Griffin, Sir Charles James Berridge Aldis and Richard Bright. They described patients with jaundice who progressed to develop confusion and died of coma. Many of them had an 'infectious cause' for jaundice, and on autopsy, they found the coverings of the brain yellow-tinged, soft and flaccid. Thus, an inaccurate perception that 'mental distress' caused jaundice was also put forth, later corrected with experiments by Friedrich Theodor von Frerichs in 1851. He found that patients who died from yellow atrophy (an old term for ALF) did not die of an increase in bile in their bodies or brains. To prove this, he injected bile into the veins of dogs. This did not reproduce the brain failure, but when ammonium carbonate was injected, the dogs developed twitching and seizures and eventually died. But this experiment was forgotten for decades until 1932, when Van Caulaert fed oral ammonia salts to patients with liver disease and found that increasing ammonia levels in blood directly resulted in brain dysfunction, and the toxic ammonia theory of hepatic encephalopathy in severe liver disease was born. Nonetheless, the term 'hepatic encephalopathy' for brain failure in patients with liver failure was coined and used for the first time only in 1957 by Dr Fazekas.

Back at the ICU, a weary Raj was updated regarding his wife's unstable condition. The only way out was immediately finding ways to get her a new liver.

'But we still don't know the cause of her liver failure,' Raj told the doctor, who was quick enough to ignore this fact.

'It does not matter,' the doctor said. 'Meera's liver has failed, and looking for a cause is not the priority.'

All that was required was to save the mother of two, which was possible only with liver transplantation, which cost approximately ₹25 lakh (or $27,000). Raj did not have that kind of money. He was already burning a hole in his pocket, and his debts with friends and family had increased. The worst part was that nobody seemed to know or care why his wife was dying. He was inside his worst nightmare: an unknown cause, a definite death and a heartbreaking loss.

Acute liver failure is a terrifying, flummoxing disease that strikes without warning. A person with a healthy liver can suddenly be fighting for life on the ventilator in ALF. The causes of ALF vary across countries. In a country like India, it is acute viral hepatitis A or E infection, while in Western countries, it is primarily due to acetaminophen or paracetamol overdose (intentional or accidental). Diagnosing ALF and identifying and treating specific causes can help reverse the liver injury or help doctors plan life-saving early liver transplantation. When jaundice, blood thinning (INR >1.5) and brain failure occur within one week, it is termed 'hyperacute ALF'; it is 'classic ALF' when the triad of symptoms occurs within two to four weeks. In the US, the diagnosis of classic ALF is considered for up to twenty-six weeks. Hyperacute ALF patients have better survival, provided the cause of liver failure is identifiable. Apart from hepatitis viruses, drugs, such as those given to combat tuberculosis, are also a frequent cause of ALF in India. In south Indian states, yellow phosphorous rat poison ingested for suicidal intent is also a common cause. However, many patients with ALF have no identifiable cause and are termed 'indeterminate ALF' or 'cryptogenic ALF'. As discussed, in Meera's case, the doctors could not find any reason for her ALF, and with only the best supportive care, Meera was inching close to death.

Transplantation was not an option for Raj.

Not now.

Until someone could figure out another option, he'd have to bleed their life savings for a high-risk procedure.

The Storm Shelter

Taking the chance, Raj decided to shift Meera to our dedicated liver-treatment facility many miles away. As a treating group that always thought out of the box, my colleagues and I knew that patients did not walk out of medical textbooks. Our treatment choice was based on evolving evidence that placed the patient at the centre. If there were questions in medical science, solutions were hidden in plain sight.

In the emergency department, I looked at the young mother and told Raj, 'My friend, she is slipping into a liver-failure-induced coma, and there seems very little we can do if we cannot protect her brain and lungs. She needs a ventilator.' Without mincing words, I reconfirmed, 'We have to keep her stable and alive to find out what is killing her.'

'Will she come off the ventilator?' Raj asked me, and I said that I did not know but assured him that it would help us buy some time to find what was failing her liver.

Raj's mother was with him, and he talked to her briefly and came back to me and said, 'Yes, please proceed to put my wife on the ventilator. Where should I sign?'

But before he filled out the documentary formalities, I told him, 'Please send your mother home with the kids. We have a long-drawn battle ahead of us.'

Complying, he approached his children, who were now inching away from the port in the storm, and told them, 'I will come home with Amma within a few days. You must go to school. Please go with grandmother and do not worry, Papa is here.'

As I heard those words, a ton of responsibility came crashing down on me. A burden that was now mine. A worry that only I was privy to, a personal dark cloud. This family of four was about to lose the most vital link in its chain, the mother, and the only thing standing between their loss and their love was my department and me.

I watched the emergency doctors readying to put Meera on the ventilator. Raj held her hand tightly before the colourless and opaque liquids were pushed into her veins to sedate her, so the doctors could place a tube into her windpipe and pump oxygen to her lungs while she slept. I watched Raj move out, giving the doctors room to complete their task. While Raj's family was missing their port in the storm, we were building them a storm shelter.

Meera was now sedated and on the ventilator. As she slept without pain or suffering, the machines provided her organs with the oxygen they required. We sacrificed our own sleep to find the cause of her acute liver injury, which, we knew, was hiding in plain sight.

Was it something we could reverse?

Could we save this young mother of two so her kids could hug her again?

The previous doctors had left no stone unturned on a thorough review of all records.

Except one.

A liver biopsy.

Since Meera was in ALF, her blood was fragile, which meant a traditional liver biopsy would possibly cause intense bleeding into her liver, which could kill her instantly. But we had another option—a transvenous biopsy, in which the liver tissue is accessed through a vein in the neck. Raj gave us consent to perform this highly complex biopsy procedure. Multiple small cylindrical cores of liver tissue were retrieved, which were rushed to the pathologist. The little liver pieces on the glass slide now held all the answers to what was killing the young woman. Tissue preparation and staining of the biopsy samples went at breakneck speed as the pathologist worked. We knew that our greatest enemy was not what was killing Meera's liver, but time itself. Meera was now showing clinical signs of increased brain swelling and pressure—the condition called cerebral edema was setting in. The chances that her brain would squeeze out of the natural holes at the base of the skull were relatively high.

~

Acute liver failure is an ancient disease that bewilders physicians to this day. Hippocratic physicians were probably the first to describe ALF during their descriptions of jaundice in the 'Hippocratic Corpus', a large body of observational evidence from ancient Greek medicine. As mentioned earlier, jaundice was considered a disease at the time, not a symptom or sign of an underlying disease. The Hippocratic physicians classified jaundice into five types. The first type, described as 'acute and rapidly fatal', is the ALF we see today. The first physicians treated ALF with a drink called 'melicrat', consisting of milk and honey, almonds, wormwood leaves and anise, further complemented with light wine and rice-gruel portions. The second type of jaundice occurred in summer (possibly viral-hepatitis-related); the third type, in winter due to 'drunkenness and chills' (possibly alcohol-associated hepatitis); the fourth type, during all seasons, due to excessive food intake (food-borne viral hepatitis); and the fifth type, mainly in winters (possibly related to other kinds of infectious hepatitis).

Modern descriptions of ALF came in the early 1800s, with observations by English physician Dr Richard Bright. Many cases described by him were probably secondary to acute viral hepatitis among the working classes in nineteenth-century London who lived in unsanitary conditions. It was not until the late nineteenth and early to mid twentieth centuries that 'epidemics of jaundice' among soldiers in war camps, especially during the Second World War, led to the appreciation that infectious causes were at the forefront of ALF. Since the infectious agents were unknown then, the disease was called 'camp jaundice' or 'jaunisse de champs'. The ALF within these cases were documented with precision, and classically described by physicians Balduin Lucké and Tracy Mallory in 1946, who called ALF 'fatal fulminant hepatitis'.

A classic case of a terrifying disease described thousands of years earlier was now lying in front of our eyes. Like the physicians at the time who were bewildered at the causes of ALF, we were struggling to find a reason behind Meera's failing liver. Since brain failure in ALF occurs due to the swelling of brain cells in the presence of high ammonia in the blood, Meera was started on a drug called mannitol.

Mannitol is an osmotic diuretic—meaning it's a drug that can increase the production of urine, thereby reducing the extra fluid that has built inside the brain. When injected into the bloodstream, mannitol ends up in the kidneys, where it cannot be reabsorbed into the blood. The mannitol within the kidneys drives out additional water and sodium from the bloodstream and excretes it in the urine. In Meera's case, this would help reduce the total brain water and brain swelling with the hope that pressures inside the skull would decrease, which would eventually help her regain consciousness. However, the increased pressure inside the skull and subsequent improvements with mannitol infusion were difficult to ascertain in a mechanically ventilated patient.

This is where generally 'bolting' would come in handy. If doctors wanted to, they could measure the pressure within the brain directly by drilling a small hole in the skull and placing a device into the brain matter—called intracranial pressure monitoring, or bolting. The critical-care doctors at my treating unit contemplated bolting Meera but decided against it because the clinical signs were suggestive of significantly high pressure inside her brain, and the risk of developing a brain bleed was concerning in her case. If the bolting resulted in a brain bleed, then everything we were fighting for would be in vain. Uncontrolled high levels of ammonia were our biggest concern. This was the sole reason for Meera's brain swelling, which would also be responsible for the brain herniation, which would kill her instantly.

Liver disease specialists at the Rigshospitalet, University of Copenhagen, in Denmark, were the first to identify the sinister aspect of ammonia in ALF conclusively. The death rate due to ALF in the 1940s to 1960s was more than 90 per cent. At the time, driven by desperation, doctors tried everything and anything they could to save patients' lives. This included the use of high-dose steroids; exchange transfusion, which involved slowly removing the patient's blood and replacing it with fresh donor blood; and sometimes even the human version of parabiosis, in which cross-circulation with another healthy human was done to help the dying liver recover and 'detox'. In some extreme cases, doctors also tried the 'ex-vivo perfusion', where the ALF patient's blood is circulated through the liver of another animal, such as a pig or primate. All these methods surprisingly failed to improve ALF or prevent death as expected.

In the early 1980s, physicians deeply concerned with the high rate of death among ALF patients started trials on a variety of treatments that came to be known as 'extracorporeal liver support devices'. In this method, external machines 'clean' toxins in the blood, much like dialysis for kidneys, giving the 'dying liver' a chance to regenerate and increase liver-transplant-free survival. Initial attempts with these machines failed miserably in saving ALF patients. But a study from Dr Fin Stolze Larsen and his team from Rigshospitalet showed that a procedure called HVPE (high-volume plasma exchange) improved transplant-free survival in the sickest ALF patients. In HVPE, a machine separates large volumes of the clear liquid part of the blood from the red blood cells, and it is discarded. Fresh, healthy plasma is mixed outside the body with the separated red blood cells and returned to the patient through another circuit. This procedure was found to have an impressive effect in reducing high ammonia in the blood. So, armed with this evidence from rigorous scientific trials, we put Meera on HVPE. In two days, after two sessions, her blood reports started to stabilize as her ammonia levels reduced. She was not worsening on the ventilator, and we found hope—a light at the end of the darkest tunnel.

~

Forty-eight hours had passed since the liver biopsy was performed on Meera, and as expected, our brilliant, wise and kind pathologist called me down to her lab. The tissue processing was completed, and the specimen was under the microscope for me to look at. I hoped, against all odds, that there was a diagnosis that we could do something about because the children were waiting for their mother back home.

'What is it?' I asked the pathologist.

'Look at it yourself ...' she told me, poker-faced.

As I peeped into the microscope, I saw bizarre things. It was like Pandora's box. All the evils unleashed together. Some areas showed features of severe fatty liver disease. Some were highly suggestive of a viral infection, while other parts showed features of autoimmune hepatitis. As I looked through into the microscope—turning the knobs and dials up and down and sideways, focusing across the whole liver tissue in low power and, at times, high magnified fields—I could even see areas of significant damage to the bile cells and bile ducts.

I turned around and looked at the pathologist and asked her, 'What am I looking at?'

'Everything you can think of,' she said worryingly. 'There is damage due to viruses, immune attack on the liver cells, damage from toxins, drugs and infections ... you name it.'

She paused, then continued, 'But we both know only one insult to the liver can mimic everything.'

'Drug-induced liver injury.'

'Time for you to find out which drug.'

I looked at her, frozen on the chair. I was exhausted.

Since Meera's arrival at our treatment centre, the only question that was repeatedly asked was regarding the use of prescription drugs, and complementary and alternative medicines. Every time, Raj had denied their use. But it was time to jump through that loop once again. This time, I would go slow, as if time had paused, and every question would be focused on shaking up and brightening Raj's brain into remembering something he might have taken for granted.

We went through the drill again. I sat down with Raj and asked him about the use of prescription drugs, herbal drugs, homeopathic remedies, medicines from traditional healers and decoctions or prescriptions from faith healers. Meera was only on thyroxine hormone supplementation for many years, which was liver safe.

Absolutely nothing came up in our conversation. Then, involuntarily and without any forethought, I asked Raj about Meera's dietary habits and recent changes to her diet. I do not know why I asked that, but it happened unexpectedly.

Raj sat up and asked, 'Does food cause liver damage?'

To which I responded, 'Yes, certain foods can cause hepatitis and liver failure—like poisonous wild mushrooms, green tea extracts and high doses of turmeric.'

'But what about protein supplements?' Raj asked me.

I was intrigued and asked him, 'What do you mean?'

Then a story started to unroll in front of me as I heard Raj go on about the central puzzle piece hidden in plain sight in this sleep-depriving, worry-fuelled story.

Two months before Meera started showing symptoms, Raj had taken her to a nearby regional fair. Meera and the children enjoyed many stores, stalls and rides. There was one particular stall that caught their attention that day. It was draped in an attractive green banner with a logo they had never seen before. The man at the counter ushered them in and told them something Meera always wanted to hear. For context, Meera was overweight because she had a low-functioning thyroid. Diet restrictions were not helping, and exercising every day was a chore. Taking care of the kids and their school activities took most of her time, and she found very little time to spare. But then there was this man in a stall, wearing a green cap and white tee with a green logo, telling her she did not have to exercise to lose weight. She only had to drink their protein shake to help her lose weight without needing the 'extra effort'.

The protein shakes were meal replacements—meaning, instead of a proper meal, one would have to drink the shakes and then depend on a water diet for long periods before having the next shake. Most consumers have only one meal daily, thinking that the shakes are taking care of their nutritional requirements. In a manner, this was a kind of ignorantly glorified starvation. And with starvation, anyone would lose weight. But this extraordinary starvation came at a price. Raj paid close to ₹10,000 (approximately $110), stretching his spending limit, for a few bottles of the protein shakes that would hardly last two months. But as instructed by the 'nutrition coach' at the counter, Meera returned home to start on the weight-loss protocol that would exempt her from physical activity.

Two months after taking the protein supplements and losing only 2–3 kg, Meera stopped overspending on the product. But then it was already too late, and a few weeks later, she started showing symptoms and signs of liver disease. I asked Raj to show me a picture of the protein supplement Meera had taken. Very keenly, he typed the letters into a Google search bar on his phone and held up the results image to my face.

At that moment, I knew we were in trouble. Meera was in a lot of trouble. We were going to fight not one terror but two. All this while, we were focused only on beating time. But suddenly, something else entered the equation.

My old friend.

Death.

This fight had just got tougher.

Drug- or toxin-induced liver injury as a cause of ALF was recognized in the late 1950s after the introduction of the anaesthetic agent called halothane. A volatile agent, halothane was given in an inhaled form to patients before surgery. Physicians at the time found that many patients developed severe hepatitis, leading to liver failure during the post-surgical period, and through close observation and study, linked it to halothane use. After halothane was removed from routine practice, the liver injury and ALF due to this drug were never again noticeable. As time passed, doctors faced another major challenge, as an epidemic of ALF cases emerged in the 1970s and 1980s. But the way ALF was managed and the role of drugs in causing ALF had changed. This time, the causative agent was a drug commonly prescribed for fever, N-acetyl-para-aminophenol, also called acetaminophen or paracetamol. In routinely recommended doses, this drug was exceptionally safe, even for those with pre-existing liver disease. However, the troubles began when it was consumed in large quantities for suicidal intent or when misused along with other liver-damaging agents, such as alcohol.

Paracetamol, when taken in extremely high doses, overwhelms detoxification pathways in the liver. Once these pathways are exhausted, a toxic byproduct called N-acetyl-p-benzoquinone imine, or NAPQI, builds up within the blood and in the liver, damaging liver cells. This ultimately leads to the loss of liver cells (a condition called necrosis) and in a very short time overwhelms the liver's ability to regenerate, leading to liver failure. A potent dose-related toxin, doctors struggled to keep patients with paracetamol-related ALF alive before a life-saving liver transplant could be offered, and many died on the transplant waitlist. But then, researchers at the King's College Hospital in London found something precious. A drug called N-acetylcysteine, or NAC, was found to replenish an antioxidant called glutathione, which helped clear the toxic NAPQI. A small but significant clinical trial in paracetamol-related ALF patients showed that it improved transplant-free survival.

The treatment of ALF due to drugs vastly changed after that. With the removal of potential liver-toxic drugs from the market and with the awareness around drug-induced liver injury leading to ALF, a significant healthcare burden was avoided. Physicians were also quick to diagnose drug or toxin-induced liver injury in their patients, which helped them initiate antidote measures, such as the use of NAC to improve survival without a liver transplant.

However, unknown to physicians at the time, a sinister cause that would become one of the biggest emerging threats to liver health and a ghastly reason for ALF was manifesting from the shadows.

Herbal and dietary supplements (HDS) are part of a larger group of substances called complementary and alternative medicines (CAMs), central to alternative medicine practice. HDS are foods defined as products taken orally that include one or a combination of vitamins, minerals, herbs, other botanicals, proteins, amino acids and sometimes organ tissues. Since HDS are not drugs, they are regulated differently from standard conventional medicines. Different types of HDS have been implicated as causes of liver injury and liver failure for decades. Single herbs and complex multiherbal mixtures are commonly identified as liver-damaging sources. Nonetheless, the presence of toxic contaminants during processing and manufacturing and intentional adulteration are also significant reasons for HDS-related liver toxicity. When there is absolutely no regulation from a safety point of view, and because HDS are treated as food supplements and not medications, every person is left to fend for themselves when it comes to severe adverse events—as in Raj and Meera's terrifying ordeal.

HDS are often used as a 'personal healthcare practice' without prescriptions from physicians or other healthcare providers. One of the earliest dietary supplements identified to cause severe liver injury was a herb known as *Larrea tridentata* (creosote bush), popularly referred to as 'chapparal'. The herb was used for its supposed antioxidant properties to improve overall health and fight weight loss, promote liver wellness as a blood purifier, improve immunity to prevent and treat cancers and HIV-AIDS infection and, finally, to slow ageing. However, like all other HDS products, none of these benefits were proven; they were only advertised as *claims* without supporting evidence. Many patients who consumed the herb in capsule form or as herbal tea landed with severe liver injury, some progressing to liver failure requiring transplantation for survival. A wide range of herbs, multiherbal products and complex HDS were, after that, identified as significant sources of severe liver injury and liver failure among consumers. Among those, one stood out as the most typical cause of herbal liver injury. The same HDS that Meera had consumed for her weight loss and that Raj had shown me on his phone: Nutrition-Club.

Nutrition-Club products are widely known to cause severe liver injury and liver failure. The National Institute of Diabetes and Digestive and Kidney Diseases, part of the US National Institutes of Health, which in turn is part of the Department of Health and Human Services, in the US, categorizes these products as a 'well-established cause of clinically apparent liver injury', based on multiple peer-reviewed clinical studies and research evidence. A recent exhaustive analysis of all case reports featuring HDS-related liver injury published between 1984 and 2021 revealed that these specific products were the most common cause of liver injury among all HDS formulations. The initial reports of liver injury were from Spain and Israel, and subsequent cases turned up in Latin America, Switzerland, Iceland and the US. In most victims, the onset was insidious, encompassing loss of appetite, fatigue, nausea and abdominal discomfort, which were followed by jaundice and the darkening of urine—all features that fit perfectly in Meera's case. The biggest challenge with HDS-related liver injury was the multiherbal aspect of the products implicated. Since multiple ingredients were present in a product, attributing the liver injury to a single identifiable toxic component was almost always difficult, and the presence of numerous known liver-poisonous agents in the products (such as green tea extracts and aloe vera) increased this challenge manifold.

Researchers from Europe had also identified in 2009 that contamination of protein supplements with the horrible bacteria *Bacillus subtilis* was responsible for liver failure in a subset of afflicted patients. This was not all. When a drug or supplement was potentially considered the cause of liver injury decades earlier, to confirm the causation, physicians performed an unthinkable act that became the gold standard for diagnosing drug-induced liver injury. Once the patient had fully recovered from the liver injury, physicians advised 'a rechallenge'—that is, the patient was asked to consume the very drug/product that was responsible for the liver injury in the first place. Once this was done, and if the patient developed liver injury again, it was confirmation that the implicated agent that had caused the severe hepatitis was indeed the drug or the product.

However, as time passed, the clinical community at large questioned the ethical aspects of this practice. What if the second time, after the rechallenge, the patient developed a severe adverse event that was not manageable with medical care? What if the patient succumbed to the rechallenge after an initial complete recovery? Considering these critical points, the rechallenge test, 'an attractive hazard', was discarded from the diagnosis of drug- or supplement-induced liver injury.

The cases of Nutrition-Club liver injury and failure were not based on correlation but on causation, because in several patients, when rechallenge was still the norm, repeat exposure to these products led to recurrence of severe HDS-related liver damage. Some patients developed such severe hepatitis after product consumption that they progressed to liver failure, which required 'super urgent' liver transplantation to preserve life. A similar pattern was also noted in our young mother of two, who was struggling to survive. Even the best medical support did not work in such situations.

It should also be mentioned that the HDS products causing liver injury and failure were not isolated to one manufacturer. Branded products from other manufacturers, such as Hydroxycut®, Move Free®,

OxyELITE Pro® and SLIMQUICK®, were also implicated, without reasonable doubt, in multiple cases of severe liver injury, some leading to death or liver transplantation.

The biggest challenge we were facing now with Meera was that most times, HDS-related severe liver injury is irreversible if it progresses to ALF. This meant that Meera would die on the ventilator without a life-saving liver transplantation. A set of clinical and laboratory criteria decides who will die without an emergency liver transplantation. In the UK, this was known as King's College Criteria. In France, they used the Beaujon-Paul Brousse or Clichy Criteria. In India, it was the ALF Early Dynamic Model, or the ALFED Model, created by gastroenterologists and hepatologists at AIIMS, New Delhi. Whichever criteria we applied, it all pointed towards Meera needing a liver transplantation, without which she would never get to see her husband, cuddle her children or gather with her family. The storm shelter we built was not proving strong enough, and the family would lose their port in the storm. I knew this because the published literature on HDS-related liver failure was depressing. The culprit components that lead to liver failure within the HDS were enigmatic. Hence, there was no antidote that we could administer, like NAC for paracetamol poisoning, to reverse the liver damage in Meera's case.

It was late in the evening, and I did not dare to meet Raj, for he was looking for a way out to get Meera back home without a liver transplant, and I was looking for ways to tell him that his beloved would never go home in the absence of one.

Heart of Darkness

'Home is where the heart is'—Pliny the Elder

Back home, I sat down with my children at the table after a warm bath. Oblivious to the burden I was carrying in my mind, they continued with their entertaining but sometimes annoying fights for dominion over the television controller. I watched my children play together around me that night, while miles away a frail grandmother watched her grandchildren sleep, waiting for their mother and father to return.

Hope is a strong force. It comes in many forms. For many, it is a prayer. For others, it is silence. And when hope gets too strong, it creates an illusion that overwhelms the natural course of an imminently dark, terminal event that deludes all logic. I kept my hopes so high that I became delusional about winning this battle for Raj and the children. Then the thought of Death entered like an equalizer. It always puts us in our place.

As a physician, I do hope. But I do not waste time praying. Instead, I use that time to think and nurture what I have studied, to put it into practical use. With Meera's case, I did not have the luxury of not spending time to think. I did not have the liberty to keep my mind at ease. That night, in bed, while everyone else slept peacefully, I lay awake, looking at the ceiling, making permutations and combinations of various medical managements for Meera.

I had to make up my mind. Do I send Meera along with Raj to a liver transplant facility, asking him to beg, borrow or steal funds to get her urgently worked up to be put on the transplant waitlist, or do I tell Raj to keep his hopes soaring high? In case of the latter, we would continue aggressive plasma exchange therapy and throw every medicine in our arsenal at Meera, which might never work, only for him to waste funds when it was inevitable that he would have to take his wife's lifeless body home. I had to choose because Raj would only do what I chose for him. My sleep that night became a formality. I wanted to speak to Raj and let him know my worries and fears about what would happen to Meera as soon as I could. I do not remember how that night passed.

In the morning, I met Raj at the medical ICU entrance. Meera was fighting on the ventilator; her liver tests were still high but had plateaued; her heart, lungs and kidneys were holding against the assault brought on by the liver failure. But we were not sure how long she could continue this fight. Her frail body was on the brink of giving up. I told

Raj that he had to beg, borrow or steal funds to get Meera better and bring her back home to their children, and that only a liver transplant would ensure that. I told him I was sorry I could not do more. Since we did not have a liver transplant programme functioning at our centre at the time, I referred Meera to the best transplant centre in the city. We shifted her quickly into an ambulance. In the ICU van, Raj sat near his mechanically ventilated wife. Along with him sat physicians and technical assistants from the ICU, who ensured Meera's safe passage to the transplant centre.

Raj leaned forward, held my right hand with both of his, lightly squeezed them, looked at me and said nothing.

Some people hope in silence.

His eyes, they thanked me. We were unsure what the future held for Raj, Meera and their cherubic little children. But now, at least now, he knew what was killing his wife. I looked back at Raj in silence, and these words filled my brain:

There is a self-referred patient for you.

The husband has previously got his sick wife discharged from multiple hospitals looking for a diagnosis. Says this place is his last hope.

I felt an ache building in my chest. I felt vulnerable, but I could not show it. I am a doctor. Doctors could not cry, even if they wanted to. So I swallowed that ache, and it went deep down inside me, into a corner of my heart where it would, from time to time, remind me of everything I let go of, trying to hold on stronger.

Raj thanked me for the diagnosis with his eyes. But his mind was morose and his heart exhausted.

'You will take her home to the children soon. All will be well,' I told him, poker-faced, with confidence I didn't feel. Raj faked a smile as the ambulance doors closed, and it drove away and disappeared into the distance.

I returned to my outpatient department, where new patients awaited me. I went into my office, sat down on my chair and stretched my legs. My mind was tired. My legs felt weak and exhausted, and the day had just begun. My sleep was the worst I had ever had, and my head hurt. I drank a tall glass of water to fill my stomach. After all, I was going to miss lunch today (like every other day) because I did not want my patients, who had travelled from cities far away, to miss their ride back or their meals, waiting for me. My body had got used to it. It complained occasionally, only to get a tall glass of water. Sometimes, I brought a piece of candy, so my blood sugar levels did not fall and my mind remained alert to listen and learn from my patients. Most of the time, I forgot my hunger when I heard the stories of my patients. As some of them were mired in despair and shrouded in sadness and hopelessness, hunger would be the last of my worries. Others were so gripping that they put me inside a clinical history that felt like a thrilling investigation, and all that excitement made my hunger feel shallow, inconsequential.

I rang the call bell on my desk, signalling the nurse to let the first patient in. A forty-year-old man named Sridhar walked in with his wife, Nayana. He was tall, strongly built and slightly balding. His face and skin were pigmented, dark and patchy. Six months back, after pointing out the darkening of his skin to his doctors, he had been diagnosed with chronic liver disease. However, he was a teetotaller and did not have a family history of liver disease. He was hard-working and sincere, and had never had to visit any hospital until then. The physician they first met with diagnosed him with high blood pressure (medically termed hypertension) and asked him to lose weight. He claimed the elevated blood pressure was the cause for the darkening of his skin.

A few months later, Sridhar felt like he was quickly forgetting things. His sleep was reversed. He felt exhausted. Even a small walk up the stairs was a chore. Every day, he woke up as if he had not slept, but returning to sleep was getting harder daily. Groggy and confused, he walked into the kitchen one day and relieved himself, thinking it was the bathroom.

Concerned and shocked, Nayana took him to a doctor in the locality, who told them Sridhar would require a liver transplant since his liver was failing.

The subsequent ammonia build-up had caused his brain to become dysfunctional. How was this even possible? It was only seven months into the diagnosis of chronic liver disease in a healthy young man, and now the doctors were advising them to go for a liver transplantation. Their world came crashing down. The couple did not have any children, and they did not have the financial support to cover the costly affair of liver transplantation. And there they were, in front of me, asking for a way out because the diagnosis was overwhelming. I looked at the reports and then at Sridhar. He was visibly in distress, physically and mentally. Just drained. There was something wrong here, not with the patient but with his diagnosis. I asked Sridhar to bring his initial tests for review and did an exhaustive clinical evaluation over the coming days.

~

The next day, while on my way to the hospital, I got a message from Raj. His nephew had voluntarily come forward to donate a part of his liver to Meera. This was great news; the recipient and donor workup and clearances were underway. I saw a ray of hope. It felt as if the clouds were passing. The liver transplant centre doctors continued the plasma exchange therapy on Meera. It helped control the ammonia levels in her body. They could keep brain death at bay with this. But time was running out. Money was still the biggest challenge. But the people from Raj's homeplace were on it, crowdfunding to save Meera's life.

For the next five days, I did not hear from Raj, and I did not have the heart to call him. What if Meera had died? What if he was coping with it and did not find time to contact me? I shook off the darkness creeping into my mind, only to face it for real.

The same evening, my phone pinged as it received a new message. It was just three words. *She is gone*. It was from Raj.

He went offline soon after.

Later, I came to know from the treating doctors at the transplant centre that the first donor did not match due to severe fatty liver disease, and that there were no immediate family members whose blood group matched for liver donation. The benefits of plasma exchange therapy had run out, and Raj had run helter-skelter trying to find altruistic donors who would come to his aid to preserve Meera's life so that he could take her to his children back home.

He had made them a promise.

A promise was a promise when it came to children. That is all they would remember—if Papa had kept his promise.

Somewhere in between all that chaos, Meera's brain had swelled and herniated through her skull, cutting off her respiration centre. As brain death ensued, her other organs started to fail when an infection hit her. Meera's heart beat as long as it could for the love of her children, but it had become weary as she battled a persistent enemy. Raj spent the final moments by the side of his brain-dead wife, sullen and silent, as she passed away into the night. Meera died on the ventilator without pain and suffering but transferred both to those surviving her.

'Every good thing must come to an end,' as the saying goes. Raj brought Meera's lifeless body back home to their children. As promised.

After Meera and Raj left, the sanctuary in my mind became a scar in the corner of my heart. I found that I could not shake off their faces from my routine. The children's faces were unforgettable. What would have gone through their minds when they saw Meera's lifeless body at their doorstep? How would they cope? How could that void be filled? How would that grief change them from the natural course of their lives?

Whenever I closed my eyes, I saw a profoundly jaundiced Meera and a melancholic Raj. I did not want to see such an ill-fated family again. One of the most critical privileges a physician possesses is the power to publish validated observations and the experience of clinical outcomes in a medical practice bound by rationale, logic and reason. A medical publication becomes evidence because it is vetted through a complex scientific peer-review system that furthers its credibility. If I was confident that Meera's death was avoidable, then that reason should be known to all, so that such tragic incidents could be averted among generally healthy people.

In August 2018, we published Meera's fatal case as a report in an influential medical journal. Our report was unique in that it was not only Meera's case that we discussed. We also sourced multiple similar products from trusted online sellers, including one sample that was retrieved from Meera's home. We then subjected them to exhaustive chemical and toxicology analysis. Our report reviewed all available published data on the same products and shed light on what was unknown to the lay public. We presented, with evidence, the analysis of unsettling data that showcased heavy-metal contamination, toxic compounds, psychotropic substances and sinister bacterial contamination in similar products, which we had purchased.

After we published the paper, our lives changed.

A Giant That Blocks the Sunlight

In late October 2019, I received a letter from a woman asking me for details of the case to prove the credibility of our published report. Since the report was peer-reviewed by scientists and clinicians who were experts in the field of drug-induced liver injury, I had very little to offer them because every pertinent detail was already in the publication. This did not satisfy her. The following communication I received was a legal letter with a threatening tone. The company claimed that my report and Meera's death were not real, and still had to be proven. They also required another confirmation from us. We had to show our 'credentials' to the infamous HDS manufacturer to prove that we were real doctors and scientists. They were on the verge of serving me a defamation notice.

The children welcomed their mother's dead body at the doorstep.

Was their sorrow a lie, a part of my imagination? Were my scars illusory?

Was Raj's grief a pretence?

How would their home be if Raj had not visited the nutritional club and Meera had not consumed that anecdotal weight-loss product? What if the whole family had decided to go for a movie that day? The children could have cuddled in their mother's arms even today.

We could not turn back time but were left to fend for the future using grief as a shield. They did not stop there. They made 'scientists' on their payroll write illogical but scathing criticisms against our report, which the medical journal published, along with a searing rebuttal from our side.

Eventually, evidence triumphed over fearmongering. When the company could not push their agenda of taking down our report through rational scientific debates—because our methods and the publication and responses to their criticism were drenched in scientific reasoning and logical rebuttals—they went radio silent. Only to come back with something we had never expected. Or faced before.

Unleashing a lot of their money power, they sent threatening legal letters to the journal's editorial board, editor-in-chief and the publisher, flexing more legal muscle in the process when rebuttals from their side beautifully failed. The legal letters were sent by a powerhouse attorney based in New Delhi. Looking to give their criticism a chance, the journal decided to put our report through another round of peer review with a new set of senior experts. Within a few weeks, the fresh peer-reviewed report ruled in our favour.

Even after a second investigational peer review that concluded that our report was credible, through more legal pressure they were successful in removing our report from all web sources and the journal. Without the consent of me and the co-authors, the journal and the publisher removed our paper from all online sources to 'satisfy' the big company and 'reduce' legal tension while making a mockery of Meera's story and her family's pain. The legal burden was too much for the journal and its editorial board to handle. Fighting a large multinational company would mean losing time and money, and as government doctors who worked in state and central institutes, they did not have either. So they took the easy way out, pushing me and my co-authors under the bus while they washed their hands of all the legal pressures. Money won and science lost. Meera's death was trivialized by the same company whose products were responsible for making her children motherless.

Everything takes a back seat when it is a fight for what is right.

A fight for our patients.

A fight for the ones who suffered.

A fight for families who had to bear the burden of being wronged.

Our report was never going to come back online. This was true. However, if we had left the decision of the journal and the publisher on our report as it was, then it would seem like Meera had never existed, her children's grief had never existed and Raj's bereavement, carrying his wife's body home, had never existed.

I ended up making more enemies out of friends.

Even though we did not win the war, we won a battle. Our paper was lost forever from online sources, away from all eyes and cast into a void. But life has different ways of giving back, which, in this case, came in the form of the Streisand effect. The Streisand effect is one where attempts to hide or censor information leads to the unintended consequence of increased awareness.

In late December 2020, an online social media user casually discussed the perils of HDS as they related to the liver. In response to that discussion, I put up facts concerning our battle with the supplement company in the context of Meera's death. This unexpectedly went viral. As responses poured in from the community—some alarmed, others plain angry—the matter was taken up by two prominent groups. I was contacted by Dr Elisabeth Bik, the renowned Dutch microbiologist and data sleuth famous for exposing over 4,000 cases of scientific fraud. A recipient of the 2021 John Maddox Prize for her relentless work in detecting image manipulation and defending research integrity, she offered me a platform to document our ordeal on her influential blog, *The Science Integrity Digest*. After Dr Bik's piece came out, the scientific and general community noticed the issues we were facing and the supplement-manufacturing giant we had been up against. The news that science lost because of money power spread like wildfire. In tandem, the people behind the powerhouse website *Retraction Watch*, a blog owned by the Center for Scientific Integrity that reports on retractions of scientific papers and related topics, took notice. After people tagged them on my post, the science writers who produced the blog, Ivan Oransky and Adam Marcus, reached out to me. They asked me to provide deep insights into how an essential study on the death of a woman was being shushed behind closed doors through threats against well-meaning doctors, scientists and public health specialists. Dr Bik and the people at *Retraction Watch* lifted the lid on the darkness that shrouded our valuable report, which was trapped in a void.

We no longer required the journal or their editorial boards' approval of scientific integrity on our paper. Real, well-meaning doctors and scientific integrity experts worldwide had ultimately endorsed our report and called out the atrocities that had happened after we published it. We felt free as our work stood tall against every attempt to tarnish it. Meera's story was back online, and the delinquent attempt at hiding its aftermath had become prime news across major social media networks.

~

Acute liver failure is a devastating disease that burdens the world. Some causes are unavoidable and accidental. But some are entirely avoidable. Herbal and dietary supplements are now a rapidly emerging reason for acute liver injury and failure among young and old. There is currently no evidence, from a clinical point of view, that these HDS are beneficial at any point in our lives. The low-level swindling by the wellness industry has affected the minds of ordinary people through promotions and advertisements. The HDS industry never keeps its promise, never gives, but only takes our hard-earned money or the people we love. A host of supplements keep getting reported from the world over in medical literature as severely liver-toxic. The typical herbal agents implicated in liver injury include aloe vera, black cohosh (or fairy candle), fenugreek, garcinia cambogia (Malabar tamarind), green tea extracts, noni fruit extracts, senna, skullcap and valerian root.

Green tea extracts are of particularly great concern here. Consuming up to three cups of standard green tea daily is relatively safe. However, green tea extracts in the form of capsule supplements or as part of multiherbal formulations are a well-documented cause of severe liver injury, liver failure requiring transplantation and even death. Green tea extracts related to liver injury and acute liver failure depend on the dose of a plant chemical component called epigallocatechin gallate or EGCG. The observed safe level of EGCG is 704 mg/day. A dose higher than this in a person who is susceptible to illness from green tea extracts causes liver injury. This risk increases in the presence of a genetic variant called HLA-B*35:01, which results in severe hepatitis, jaundice and liver failure. The usual intake of green tea from natural tea infusions is 10 g, which contains 75 mg of EGCG. However, herbal supplements or multi-ingredient products could contain an EGCG consumption equivalent ranging from 125–900 mg/day, with a very high risk of developing liver injury and failure. After the European Food Safety Authority concluded that consumption of EGCG exceeding 704 mg per day might increase the likelihood of liver damage when taken as a food supplement, new legislation in the European Union set new labelling requirements, restricting the amount of green tea extract.

Our report on the Nutrition-Club product was the first from the Asian continent. Doctors and researchers across the world have published cases of similar liver injuries, and I would discuss them on my social media. Feeling the intense heat of logical criticism and unable to make scientific rebuttals against any of my posts, the company went ahead and did something more drastic. This time, they sent me a 'Cease and Desist' notice asking me to sign an affidavit their lawyers had prepared. It was an excellent little pre-made template document of two pages, essentially asking me to sell my heart and soul to the Devil. The affidavit and the 'Cease and Desist' notification found their way to my email bin soon after.

Early the following year in 2021, I received a call from a reporter for *The New York Times*. She wanted to run Meera's story, pieces on my ordeal and the roller-coaster ride of publishing the report, and an interview with Raj. Two years after Raj's heartbreaking three-word message, I finally called him. Being featured in *The New York Times* was an ample opportunity for me and my work, and for others to learn from Meera and Raj's story. Raj had found a new job and moved to a new place. I asked him about the children.

'They are busy with school and studies,' he said. 'But they miss their mother every day.'

The reporter had travelled to Kochi to meet me. She was sweet and well-meaning. I asked Raj if he would be kind enough to speak with her regarding the past. He paused for a minute and complied. He complied because he considered me family. He did not want to relive it again and agreed to it only for me. The two met soon after, and the reporter spoke to Raj with the help of a translator.

I called Raj that evening and asked him how it went. His voice broke. He had to relive that gloom and did it for me because he could never forget me. After all, I had found out what was killing his wife, even though I could not get her better. Getting featured in *The New York Times* was a great opportunity. People would know about me and my work. But was this a selfish endeavour or did I want Meera's story to be heard? Two things would happen: I would be in the limelight, and awareness of the

HDS industry and their transgressions would come to light; but at the expense of digging up another man's dark, tear-filled past.

Raj told me one thing during that call, and it hit me hard. He said he remembered Meera ever so painfully only when he visited hospitals or thought of me. Over the phone, his voice kept breaking, and I felt his sobs inside.

I felt miserable. So I talked to *The New York Times* reporter the following day and lied to her that many things that were possible from my side were impossible due to various technical reasons. And we called it off. I knew that *The New York Times* had a multitiered fact-checking system, and Raj would have to relive his tragedy repeatedly. Again and again. It was not worth it. My highlight in *The New York Times* was not worth another man reliving his burdened past.

During our last conversation, I thanked Raj and told him that *The New York Times* story was called off and that he could call me anytime for help, advice or opinions. I was there for him and wanted nothing from him, but he could ask for anything from me.

The Dalai Lama once said, 'Compassion is the wish to see others free from suffering.'

I have not spoken to Raj since that call.

Meera remains in the corner of our hearts—a scar in mine, a fire in his.

Raj has not had to relive that pain because of me ever since.

I do not call him.

Not anymore.

~

A couple of days later, I got a call from my department staff as I was getting into the car to go home after a long day's outpatient review work. Sridhar had come for admission, and his wife insisted that he get admitted as soon as possible. I asked my staff to give Nayana the phone to see why they needed immediate admission through the now-closed outpatient department. Sridhar's legs had swelled up fast, and he had got confused about the bathroom again. He had walked into the living room in a daze. She was palpably worried for her husband and felt that he would be safer inside a hospital than in their own home. As a couple without children, they only had each other. The loss of one would devastate the other.

Losing the closest family member leaves a void that can never be filled. Even if we try to fill it with good memories, paradoxically, the void only gets bigger until you run out of memories, and the looped memories drag you down and drown you. Then the loss takes over until time restores the balance through meaningful distractions that come after.

I spoke with Nayana and directed them to the emergency department so that Sridhar could be admitted as soon as possible. I then called the duty doctor in the emergency department to brief him about Sridhar.

'Oh! I was just about to call you, sir,' he told me.

'Why, is there a consult?' I asked.

'Not a consult, sir, but an admission under you to the medical ICU.'

'But I did not get any notification about a possible referral from another hospital,' I told him.

'He is only thirty-one years old and in a coma. He is already on the ventilator, and we have stabilized him to be shifted to intensive care,' the young doctor told me, uneasy.

'Is it awful?' I asked him, concerned.

'Sir, looks like it is a case of acute-on-chronic liver failure. The wife is young, they have no children, and she is wailing here, asking us to get him better for them to live long and have children. I do not know what to tell her.'

I sensed it. The hair at the back of my neck stood up. I already had Sridhar on my mind. But now someone else, a much younger man, battling one of the most horrendous medical syndromes known to humankind, had landed at my doorstep, looking for sanctuary. I did not have one but two childless couples to care for. I needed all the rest I could to focus all my energy on these two men.

The death of my patients had drained me over the past few years, and I was reduced to a burning candle dripping away while trying to light everything up—for those around me and myself. I looked forward to getting back home—seeing my children, holding them, easing my heart, seeing my wife's smile—and feeling lighter, melting my worries, gathering focus, to fight not one but two battles ahead.

Back home, I entered the bathroom, locked the door behind me and stepped into the shower.

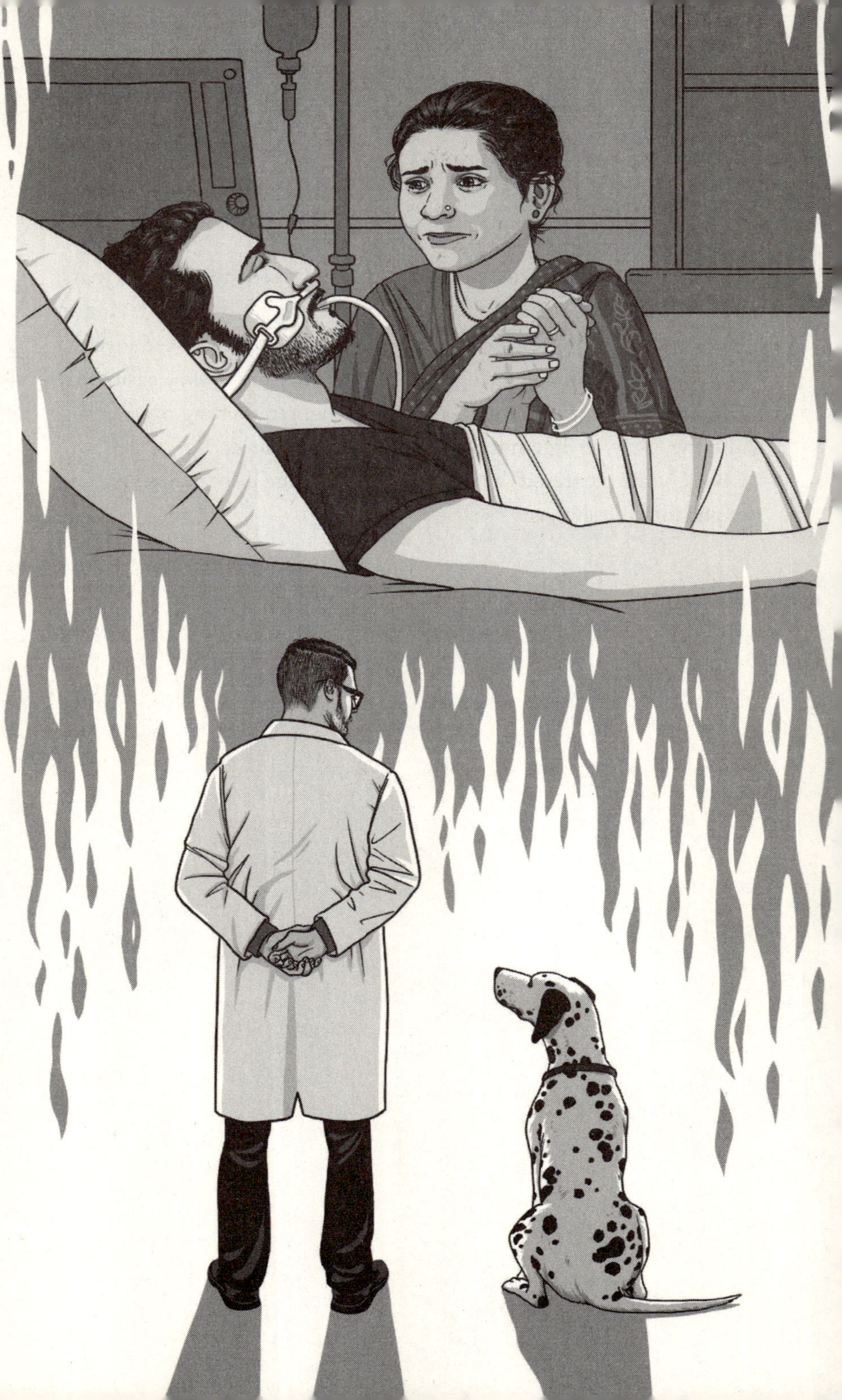

CHAPTER 2

Lo and Behold, the Canopic Jar of Imset

Comprehension of Chronic Liver Disease and Its Complications

Juniper's Last Whimper

'Death is the sound of distant thunder at a picnic.'
—W.H. AUDEN

Please Don't Go

I MUST TAKE YOU TO ANOTHER PLACE TO UNDERSTAND WHAT was coming next. It is a small place within my heart—a place where I learnt to understand humanism and the sadness of unexpected loss; not through humans but through a dog.

I have a simple and satisfying life. Loving, caring parents who gave me the best education I could have—my father, who spoke so little, but when he did speak, he guided me across confusing junctures in my life; and my mother, who unconditionally supported my decisions. I have a brother and two sisters who complete my ordinary life, and I have them all with me. Then came Teena, my beloved, and our children. I had never felt the kind of happiness I do when they are around me. Life was good. All of us, here, together, now.

When I saw Death guide my patients away from their families, I could not, at first, fathom the depth of that loss. I would imagine losing a sibling, I would imagine losing a parent—but it would all end with a mild heartache that I could shake off. I had never actually felt a loss.

And then Juniper came into my life. Juniper became ours in 2018, when I saw her inside a small pet shop for the first time, looking at me from her medium-sized cage while my car was at a stop signal. The signal turned green, and I quickly left the spot, but a part of me stayed behind at that junction, looking at that cute little Dalmatian puppy. I went home and told my mother and younger sister that I had seen the sweetest dog. Before we knew it, I was back at the signal junction, but this time, inside the shop. I bought that little puppy and got her home to be with us. I named her after the bittersweet, award-winning episode 4 in the third season of the massively popular television series *Black Mirror*. The episode's name was 'San Junipero', and it broke my heart, pleasantness interspersed with regret, the notion that life with a dog, and then without it, felt the same.

Juniper, or Joony, as we called her, was part of everything at our home from the first day onwards. She could never be alone—either she had to be around us, or we had to ensure that we were around her! We were a unit. She was never detached from us and was closest to me because I was the first to see her. Sometimes, I thought she was a caring human trapped inside a dog's body. She would show love, regret, sadness and loneliness, depending on our presence and interactions with her.

Juniper grew with our family—sharing in our joys, mischief, and everyday rituals—with a loyalty and gentleness that made her my children's dearest friend. Whether sneaking chocolates with them at night, lining up for a scolding after some shared mischief or patiently waiting for scraps from our breakfast plates, she was always part of us—never demanding, always giving. Even when ignored in the flurry of play, she bore it with quiet grace, teaching me more about patience and unconditional love than any human ever has. She found happiness simply by being near us—snuggled between us during board games, watching us watch TV and content with an empty cone even if there was no ice cream. In a world where presence is often transactional, Juniper reminded us what it meant to truly belong, to care without expectation, and to love without judgement.

A year after we got Joony, she gave us something so beautiful, little parts of her: eight puppies, or little 'Joonies', as I called them, running helter-skelter in our house. Everywhere we looked, we saw her in her puppies. Eight spongy little bundles of joy. Since we could not take care of all of them, we had to give away five to other caring families. But like a patient mother, Juniper cared for all of them, and let us play with them and cuddle them without possessiveness.

My children adored the puppies, and together with Juniper, they filled our home with love and care. Despite having her own puppies, Juniper always chose to be near my children—her first loves—having grown up with them, played in their imaginary worlds, and stayed close when they were unwell. Her eyes reflected sorrow when they were sick, and her love for us was so deep, so unconditional, it often made me question if we were even capable of loving her back the same way. Unlike us, dogs don't complicate love—they just give it, freely and without conditions or judgements. Some moments—like the joyful chaos of our treat-circle games, where Juniper and her pups playfully fought for airborne snacks—were pure magic. They were reminders that for them, being near their humans was everything.

Then one day, Juniper was eating less and was inactive for a day. By afternoon, she was breathless. I was at the hospital, looking after my patients and taking care of their concerns while my best friend was struggling at home. When she became blue, my mother rushed her to a nearby pet clinic, where they gave her high-flow oxygen to keep her brain functioning. The veterinary doctors found that her lungs were filled with fluid because her heart was not beating well, and it was slowing down. The pump that filled her body with all the blood she needed to keep her brain working was failing because of a severe viral infection. Her heart rate was off the charts and was going haywire. In an acute heart failure stage, the doctors put her on everything they could, and she seemed to stabilize. My mind was disturbed while caring for patients at the hospital. I tried hard not to focus on what Juniper was going through, all alone in the corner of that pet clinic, trying to breathe in all that oxygen without losing consciousness so that she could see her favourite humans around her at some point. When the hospital work finished, I rushed to the pet clinic to see Juniper. It was almost night, and the moment she saw me, her eyes lit up, and whatever energy was left in her was used for just one thing—she wagged her tail even when she was utterly breathless.

No words were spoken, but it was everything she could tell me then.

I went close to her, held her face in my hands and hugged it, and called her name out. She kept wagging her tail, and with all the energy she could muster let out a distressing cry—something between a howl and a whimper that came from beyond—that I will never forget until I die.

It felt like she knew.

It felt as if she knew she would not see me again.

But I was not letting go. I was hopeful.

We try our best. We do it for everyone.

We do it for strangers who come as patients. We are masters of medical science.

This was our playground.

Death was passing. We were here to stay and fight.

Overnight, Juniper survived, and I felt more hopeful.

We are going to get through this, I thought.

~

In the morning, when I spoke to the doctor, she told me Juniper was holding on.

It was not a good day for me. I had to leave for Chennai to speak at an event where I was invited by the Indian Society of Gastroenterology,

Tamil Nadu State Chapter. I had two long sessions to complete. It was Saturday, and I would be back only the following afternoon. On my way to the airport, just as we reached near the clinic where Juniper was admitted, my phone showed me an ad on Instagram featuring a Dalmatian. I could not explain why that happened, but it made me uneasy. I asked my driver to turn the car towards the pet hospital. I would be late to the airport, but I had to squeeze in the time somehow. I wanted to see Juniper.

Somehow, I felt that she wanted to see me too. When I entered the admissions room, I saw something that would stay with me forever. I saw the duty doctor and a nurse giving chest compressions to Juniper. She had gone into a cardiac arrest a few minutes before—probably around the same time I saw the advertisement on my phone and decided to take the detour. I had seen enough deaths in the hospital—from my bachelor's training until my current professional life—so many deaths that would numb a human, that I knew that Juniper had died. Her longing eyes were now fully dilated and lifeless, and she was not breathing. I joined the vet and the nurse in giving Juniper more chest compressions as we tried to put a breathing tube into her windpipe to get in as much oxygen as we could. Finally, a nurse got the tube in, and we bagged her lungs full of oxygen.

But she would not wake up.

She lay limp in my arms as I kept the compressions going on. I kept working on her, hoping that she would come back and I could take her home. But she did not. I kissed her tightly on her long face (twice, just like she always loved) and cried out, in my head, *Please don't go*.

But she was already long gone. I stepped away from her limp body, looking one last time at what was left of all that love packaged into flesh and bones, while the doctor declared the time of her death.

Do you know how it feels when a good old friend passes away?

Do you know how it feels when it happens in your arms?

Do you know how it feels when it is family?

I got into my car and noticed that my driver knew Juniper was no longer alive by looking at my face.

I looked like Death itself. Throughout the journey to the airport, I kept my face impassive, and my eyes closed. I did not want my driver to see me cry. Then the phone rang. Teena knew that Juniper was no more and had called to check on me. But I told her I did not want to speak because I would wail on the phone, and my driver would see me in my most vulnerable state. So she ended the call, and I reached the airport in forty minutes.

I got through the main gate, got my boarding pass from the kiosk, pulled my baggage across the floor, got into the elevator and completed my security check, where the officer, seeing my face, asked me if I was sick. I told him I was not, that it was just a headache due to lack of sleep, and he let me go. I got to the boarding area and saw that Gate 1 was empty. My boarding was from Gate 4. But I went to Gate 1 and—sitting behind a corner, huddling, away from all eyes—burst into tears. I had to release it. I had to release as much as possible so I would not do this inside the plane. I somehow gathered myself up from the chair, went to the rest room and washed my face of the tears. It seemed like forever because I could not stop them from streaming down my face.

Composing myself, I returned to my gate just in time for the announcement that boarding had commenced. I sat like a stuffed toy on the flight—unemotional, non-interactive. I put on my headphones and listened to music; a distraction stored offline on my phone until I reached my destination. The first song played was Alan Walker's piano rendition of 'Faded'. I wanted to stop it then and there, but it overwhelmed me, and I closed my eyes and listened to it on loop until I deplaned. I love to hate that song now. It reminds me of a difficult day, but also of the day when I was with Juniper when she left me. I guess we all have a song like that.

For the rest of the day, I spent time with doctors at the meeting discussing medical topics, all the while closely packing in all my grief and wandering thoughts into a corner of my heart, somehow getting through my presentations. It was late evening, and I only wanted to go to my hotel room. I ate a bit at the dinner and told my hosts that I had an early flight to catch and wanted to retire early to bed.

After saying my goodbyes, I rushed to my room, closed the door and crashed on the soft chair. I cried my heart out again and again until I unknowingly drifted to sleep, only to be woken up by the phone ringing. I got up groggily and saw that it was Teena, likely worried that I had not called her since I had landed. I apologized for my forgetfulness and told her I wanted to finish the day; somehow, I had missed all her calls. She knew how I felt and asked me how I was. I was sobbing intermittently and told her that all the tears that I shed and the amount of time I spent crying was not helping me. However much I cried, I was unable to satisfy that hungry ache inside my chest.

Unable to satiate the sadness, I slept off into the night, thinking about days bygone and those ahead. We think that 'grief slowly gets smaller with time', but in reality 'grief stays the same, but life slowly grows bigger around it'.

In a country where life-saving healthcare is unaffordable for most humans, Juniper never stood a real chance. This is a place where families must choose between saving their children's future or keeping a loved one on a ventilator. Where even humans lose the battle, not because of disease but because of poverty and inequality, what hope did my dog have? If human lives are priced out, how could Juniper possibly survive?

What I learnt from losing her was that regret is brutally honest. It arrives too late, teaches too much and lingers longer than grief itself. Regret is the true equalizer—it seeps into every quiet moment and haunts every pause. I realized that the present matters more than any plan or dream. Time doesn't heal, it just moves on while we remain stuck. We don't recover, we adapt. And in that adaptation, I learnt to value time over money.

The night before she died, Juniper was alone in a room full of unfamiliar dogs and strangers. I, who had raised her from a pup, was home with my family, thinking of her only in spare moments. I imagined myself in her place—dying in a sterile ICU, surrounded not by loved ones, but by strangers in scrubs. That thought broke me. Would I ever make peace with my regrets about Juniper? Could I ever forgive myself for not being there when she needed me most?

What did Juniper feel the night she died, and the morning before? I was there—but only to bag oxygen into her lifeless lungs. I was too late to her death, just as I had often been too late in her life. Too late to show her how much I truly cared, how deeply I loved her.

What did she see in those final moments? Surrounded by people, yet still utterly alone. I think about that constantly. I would give anything to go back—to be there beside her, holding her as she slipped away. Even if I couldn't stop her from going, I wish the last thing she saw was me, the one who brought her home. I wish the last thing she felt was my hand on her cold fur. That would have meant everything—to her and to me. To let her die feeling loved. Because to die in love is a great thing of beauty.

When it is time for you to say goodbye to your family, or when it is time for a dear one to say goodbye to you, the time invested in making memories will eclipse everything else. Juniper's loss taught me that.

In my best friend's death, I found a deeper meaning in my family than I had ever imagined. And in my patients. And their families.

Losing Juniper left me numb and emotionally drained. If the death of a pet could feel this devastating, I couldn't begin to imagine the pain of losing a beloved person—a child, a partner, a parent. Her death gave me a glimpse into the depth of sorrow families endure when a loved one is sick or dying.

Some may dismiss it and say Juniper was just a dog. But she wasn't. She was a true friend, my family, and losing her was unlike anything I've ever experienced. With her, there was no judgement, no expectations—just silence, patience and reflection. That kind of companionship is rare, even among humans. I once thought witnessing death would harden me, make me resilient. But it never did. Each loss, including hers, breaks me all over again.

Juniper is irreplaceable, but she left behind little parts of herself in those who still love us, and we will love them in return. I'll carry her in my heart and in a song—forever. In quiet moments, I'll keep whispering to her: 'Thank you for all the love, my friend. I'm sorry I couldn't save you or be there when you needed me most.'

Loving Dogs and Dying Men

Harish was sedated and on the ventilator. While the drugs and relaxants kept him comfortable, the beeping, huffing and puffing machines hooked into his windpipe bathed his organs with the medicines and oxygen required to keep him alive. His wife, Nalini, was outside the ICU, waiting for my update. I looked through the clinical charts with attentiveness. Harish was an obese man. He had uncontrolled diabetes, and was very irregular with his medications and meal timings.

As a young man thrust into the family business, he worked hard to improve on what his father had done before him. Work was his life, and everything else became secondary. As part of business meetings, Harish often travelled and hosted parties for clients where he would enjoy a drink or two, and sometimes more. In recent months, he had adopted a strange pattern of alcohol use: binge-drinking. For a typical adult male, this pattern corresponds to consuming five or more drinks (four or more drinks in an adult female) in about two hours. With such excessive drinking, his liver was persistently affected by the inflammation brought on by alcohol. Since he was obese, with uncontrolled diabetes and unrestricted and untimely dietary behaviour, he had a pre-existing medical condition: chronic liver disease related to fatty liver.

The knowledge that fatty liver was associated with alcohol and tuberculosis infection (due to poor nutrition) was first identified by the English physician Thomas Addison in 1836. Cecil Watson, a physician from the US, first reported the finding of a 'greasy' liver on anatomical evaluation in 1842. But it was only later, in 1938, that the American pathologist Charles Connor described a man with long-standing fatty liver who developed liver scarring, leading to chronic liver disease and eventually cirrhosis. When fat accumulates in the liver, it produces chemicals that cause swelling and damage to liver cells, where scar tissue forms as part of the healing. This is called fibrosis. When fibrosis progresses, it eventually results in the loss of liver cells and lack of liver regenerative capacity, leading to well-developed scars surrounding nodules made of the remaining functioning liver cells, which is termed cirrhosis.

Harish's liver was already weak and chronically damaged, and the additional alcohol binges landed him in a state of liver failure. This condition, when an acute insult (or a stressor) suddenly destabilizes a chronically weakened organ, making it ready to call it quits, is also known as acute-on-chronic liver failure, in short, ACLF.

To diagnose cirrhosis, a host of blood tests and imaging are required. Blood investigations will show low platelet count and albumin levels (a protein produced by the liver found in blood) and imaging will show a coarse liver with an irregular surface or nodule formation. In some cases, it appears shrunken. The spleen, an organ of extreme immune functions situated on the left upper abdominal region below the lungs, separated by the thick muscles of the diaphragm, will increase in size—a condition called splenomegaly. Some patients showcase the features associated with high liver pressures: such as fluid in the abdomen (ascites) and large dilated veins in the food pipe, stomach and abdomen, called varices or collateral veins. Not all liver diseases lead to a shrunken liver. Sometimes, the liver size may be normal or even enlarged, even in cirrhosis. The gold standard for diagnosing chronic liver disease—or the end stage of its spectrum, cirrhosis—is to perform a liver biopsy. The biopsy will show thick scars surrounding nodules made up of whatever liver cells are left after the ongoing damage—in general, the pathologists would call this 'a cirrhotic pattern'.

Back in the inpatient room, Sridhar and Nayana were waiting for me to update them about our plans for them. Sridhar had not slept well the previous night, and even after falling asleep, he could not remain so for more than a couple of hours. It was less than eight months since the diagnosis of chronic liver disease in Sridhar, and he was showing the symptoms and signs of advanced liver disease—along with those of hepatic encephalopathy, which we have explored in greater detail in chapter 1. But there was something amiss.

Sridhar's baseline investigations by my radiology colleagues revealed that his liver was normal in size and shape. The blood panel revealed low platelet counts, but the liver tests showed normal albumin levels and advanced clinical features of cirrhosis were not very evident. This was indeed strange because, without the classic features of cirrhosis, it was surprising that Sridhar would be affected by encephalopathy. However, there was a group of conditions that could mimic advanced liver disease in its absence. For us to get 'a diagnosis' we had to take Sridhar through a series of protocol-based tests that would help eliminate multiple causes that stood between us and his diagnosis.

Chronic liver disease is the general term that doctors use interchangeably with cirrhosis. But, as I discussed earlier, the latter is the end of the spectrum of the former. As cirrhosis progresses, the scar tissue increases and the residual liver cells die out. Increased scar tissue leads to an increase in the pressure inside the liver as the organ stiffens. This increase in liver pressure can be reflected by various measurable factors, clinical and investigational. Once the pressure starts increasing beyond a certain point, the large vessel supplying blood to the liver, the portal vein, increases in size and dilates (widens). This increase in liver pressure, as you may recall from the prologue, is known as portal hypertension. Once portal hypertension progresses, larger vessels, collateral veins, and even bigger ones called shunts (when the collateral vein diameter goes above 8 mm) develop. Portal hypertension usually develops with the progression of chronic liver disease to cirrhosis. The hope is that the disease will be caught before getting to that stage.

The first step in identifying chronic liver disease is to look at the liver function tests. The tests may or may not be abnormal (subtle or otherwise) early on and in advanced liver disease. The reasoning that a normal liver function test equates to a 'healthy' liver is wrong. More extensive investigational tools, such as contrast-enhanced computed tomography (CT) and magnetic resonance imaging (MRI) scans, are not sensitive enough to diagnose early chronic liver disease. However, they can quickly identify advanced cirrhosis and features of portal hypertension.

Another non-invasive test is usually performed to identify chronic liver disease. In 2003, Laurent Sandrin of the Echosens company in France published a novel diagnostic technique using ultrasound to assess liver stiffness or the magnitude of scarring in the liver at the bedside. In this test, ultrasonic waves are passed into the liver using a probe placed on the abdomen surface. The speed at which the waves are received back is used to map the stiffness inside the liver. The stiffer the liver, the faster the waves bounce back to the receiver on the probe. This became popularly known as the FibroScan® test, and it's widely used to diagnose cirrhosis without the need for a liver biopsy. FibroScan® test values below 6 kPa (kilopascals) are considered healthy for a liver.

A newer generation of this test is called the shear-wave elastography, which can be done under real-time ultrasound conditions and takes less time to complete. The higher the values on these tests, the greater the chance of an underlying chronic liver disease or cirrhosis.

In patients who are diagnosed with cirrhosis, the disease progresses through various stages of complications. It was Mary Ann Payne and George Wantz who, in 1961, described and proposed a scoring system that could reliably provide information on the stages of cirrhosis, taking into consideration various complications to predict outcomes, called the Wantz–Payne score. In 1964, a surgeon at the University of Michigan, Dr Charles Gardner Child III, and his general surgery student, Jeremiah Turcotte, copied the Wantz–Payne scoring system (without attribution) to classify stages of cirrhosis in their review. After almost a decade, in 1972, the system, which is currently widely known as Child–Turcotte staging, was modified to a better one by clinical epidemiologist R. Nicholas Pugh. The modified system, which included five investigational variables—the presence and severity of brain dysfunction and fluid in the abdomen; and the levels of total bilirubin, albumin and bleeding risk (identified by the prothrombin time on blood tests)—came to be known as the Child–Turcotte–Pugh (CTP) classification or more commonly as Child staging of cirrhosis. It categorized patients into groups on the basis of scores (Class A, 5–6; B, 7–9; and C, 10–15). Unstable patients were under Classes B and C, and the ones who realistically required liver transplantation to survive longer were placed in Class C.

With this knowledge in hand, we subjected Sridhar to clinical and investigational tests to confirm chronic liver disease and high liver pressure. His liver stiffness and function tests were normal, except for low albumin. His ultrasound, however, showed something strange: the presence of collaterals around the liver. A CT scan was ordered.

While we waited for the CT reports, I received a notification from the ICU that Harish's condition was getting worse. His disease, the syndrome of ACLF, was rapidly progressing. On the ventilator, his kidneys were slowly shutting down, the kidney function tests were skyrocketing and urine output was reducing by the hour. His liver was conclusively cirrhotic, confirmed on a bedside ultrasound scan that showed a shrunken liver, large spleen and fluid in the abdomen. Along with severe jaundice and brain failure, and now failing kidneys, Harish had entered the realm of multiple organ failure. The onset of multiple organ failure in a patient with ACLF meant only one thing. It was time for the family and patient to meet the doctors' old friend, Death.

But the art of clinical medicine is not about giving up. As mentioned in the prologue, doctors are inherently teachers—they teach patients and their families to sail across trials and tribulations that could eventually end with death, or they teach themselves to cope with the expected, or unexpected, but heartbreaking loss of a patient and learn from it. Moreover, they know to never sit on their laurels in their practice. But they are also teachers of a different kind. They must teach themselves when to let go and when to keep fighting for a patient. Choosing to let go is not an act of abandonment or losing ourselves in the unknown. Instead, it represents the profound internal strength required to release our grip on a situation that is fading away—no matter how desperately we wish to save it. Sometimes, clinical medicine is a fight for comfort, not a win. Even in the advanced stages of ACLF, clinical practice is strengthened with a pragmatic approach that keeps the patient at the centre: the clinical algorithm.

Acute-on-chronic liver failure—the concept of an acute event destabilizing a stable, known or unknown pre-existing liver disease—was first put forth by Japanese researchers in 1995. In their original report, they described patients with heavy alcohol consumption in whom the underlying stable cirrhosis became unstable due to the presence of severe alcohol-associated hepatitis, leading to jaundice, brain failure, fluid in the abdomen and rapid onset of various other organ failures. This resulted in a high death rate within a month, in the absence of liver transplantation. Decades later, multiple clinical societies that worked for the betterment of liver disease patients, including the European Association for the Study of Liver, described various stages of ACLF, which helped doctors make critical decisions on patient management. Patients were stratified into ACLF Classes 1 to 3, depending on the number of organ failures. Compared to those with no organ failures, ACLF patients with more than three organ failures had a death rate approaching 90 per cent at the end of one month.

Harish was in ACLF Class 3, and his death was imminent. The number of patients with ACLF and more than three organ failures surviving without a liver transplant at six months was zero. In such patients, the logical option was to withdraw care that would drain financial resources and continue comfort care to provide the patient with a dignified death.

But Harish was so young, and withdrawing care was a difficult decision for me to make, even when the medical science evidence fed my brain contrasting data. If I faced so much difficulty in deciding on medical care in this situation, I could not imagine how the family would ever make that decision for their loved one, leaving their beloved to die on the ventilator. After discussing this with his young wife, we decided to try everything possible to give Harish a fighting chance. After all, when patients could not fight for themselves, we had to take up that fight and not let go at the outset. So we put Harish on a special treatment called plasma exchange therapy.

~

In the ancient history of medicine, approximately 3,000 years ago, Egyptian physicians initially practised bloodletting as a treatment option for various illnesses. As this practice spread to Greece and Rome and later to the Arab world and Asia, various pre-scientific era theories made in support of this practice originated. The most important of them was from ancient Greek medicine, from the Father of Modern Medicine, Hippocrates (whom we discussed in the prologue; 460–370 BCE), which was later enhanced by Galen of Pergamum (129–216 CE). This dubious practice, according to the ancient Greeks, was based on the irrational thought that the human body was made up of four basic elements (earth, air, fire and water) which manifest as basic 'humours' in the body: blood, phlegm, black bile and yellow bile. They proposed that diseases occurred when there was an imbalance among these humours. When the disease condition was closely related to the blood humour, also known as a sanguine type of disorder, then letting out the 'bad blood' was supposedly considered effective in improving the patient's condition. This was an illogical thought, but the pre-scientific-era therapeutics were mostly based on observations and beliefs rather than testability, evidence and reliability.

In the current era, Indian Ayurvedic practitioners still follow various forms of bloodletting to treat diseases from infections to diabetes and even neurodevelopmental disorders (such as autism), stuck in impractical knowledge that is a remnant of a bygone era. Ayurvedic bloodletting, or Raktamokshana, involves several specialized techniques to extract 'bad blood'. This includes suction via animal horns (Shrunga) or vacuum-sealed bottle gourds (Alabu), localized skin scraping (Pracchana) and direct vein-puncturing or cutting-through methods like Siravyadha and Suchi Avacharana, as well as the application of Ghatiyantra (cupping) and medicinal leeches (Jalauka).

Bloodletting was still considered a valid treatment in the seventeenth century, until new scientific methods appeared, conclusive descriptions of clinical anatomy and human physiology were made, the pathological and physiological mechanisms of disease development and progression were identified, and more effective diagnostic tools evolved. Bloodletting, currently known as phlebotomy, has been reduced to indicated use in only three major conditions clinically, which have nothing to do with the 'humour theory'.

Today, phlebotomy is used as an adjunct therapy for treating diseases such as hemochromatosis (a genetic disorder in which iron builds up in the body and the intermittent removal of excess iron reduces iron-induced organ damage); polycythemia vera (a bone marrow disorder leading to overproduction of red blood cells, and the removal of excess blood helps reduce red cell mass and decreases the risk of dangerous blood clots in the brain, heart, lungs and other major organs); and finally, porphyria cutanea tarda (a group of genetic diseases that results in abnormal heme, an iron-containing compound that forms part of haemoglobin and helps bind oxygen by red blood cells, and iron metabolism leading to iron accumulation and toxicity in various organs).

Scientific progress and the understanding of blood removal, especially the removal of specific blood components to treat multiple illnesses, came from the sceptical practice of ancient bloodletting. Whole blood contains multiple types of cells as well as a liquid fraction. The liquid fraction, called plasma, comprises water, proteins, wastes and toxins derived from metabolism; minerals; clotting factors; and immune-system-associated proteins called immunoglobulins.

Plasmapheresis means removal of the plasma fraction from the blood using a specific machine through central (a large main internal vein easily accessed from outside—for example, a femoral vein) or peripheral (a small, easily accessible surface vein—for example, a brachial vein) venous access. The plasma removal technique on small animals was first described by Russian scientists Vadim Yurevich and Nikolay Rosenberg of the Imperial Medical and Surgical Academy of St. Petersburg in 1913. However, it was made effectively popular, and the term 'plasmapheresis' was coined by Dr John Abel and his colleague Leonard Rowntree of Johns Hopkins Hospital in 1914 through multiple animal experiments.

When plasmapheresis was associated with the provision of replacement with blood products after plasma removal, it was called plasma exchange. Even though various safer techniques to therapeutically remove plasma from humans emerged in the late 1950s, the clinical utility of plasma exchange as a standard treatment was identified only in the 1960s, after Dr Michael Rubinstein used the method to remove life-threatening antibodies from the blood of a young man with an autoimmune disease. This disease, known as thrombotic thrombocytopenic purpura, affected the platelets, leading to life-threatening bleeding.

Plasma exchange became popular for the treatment of various diseases, especially autoimmune disorders, and for managing toxin-induced organ injuries, such as rat poison (zinc phosphide) ingestion. Decades later, the utility of plasma exchange as a viable option for stabilizing patients with acute liver failure and ACLF emerged. The idea was that the removal of 'bad' plasma, rich in toxins that had built up in the body because a failing liver could not handle it, and its replacement with fresh 'good' plasma would improve clinical outcomes.

In Harish's case, we deeply hoped that plasma exchange, along with kidney support in the form of dialysis, would help us downstage the ACLF so that we could offer him a definitive treatment option, such as curative liver transplantation.

~

While Harish was stabilized on the procedures, we revisited Sridhar's final test reports. After the initiation of ammonia-lowering therapies, his memory disorders and sleep patterns had drastically improved. However, the CT imaging showed something very sinister. A large abnormal blood vessel, a venous shunt over 3.5 cm in diameter, had formed inside his abdomen, along with an enlarged spleen, in the absence of any evidence of cirrhosis. We immediately knew where this was going. Sridhar had features of portal hypertension, or high liver pressures, in the form of large abnormal vessels (called collaterals) and a large shunt and enlarged spleen with low platelet count, but in the absence of pre-existing liver disease. This condition, a rare diagnosis in which liver pressures are seemingly elevated in the absence of cirrhosis, is called non-cirrhotic portal hypertension, or NCPH. On the one hand, we were fighting for Harish, who was facing the terrifying stage of cirrhosis, and on the other hand, with Sridhar, we were grappling with the management of the extreme clinical consequences of NCPH.

Fright, Flight or Fight

Non-cirrhotic portal hypertension is a group of disorders in which the blood vessels, mainly the veins of the liver, are affected to varying degrees of damage, resulting in features associated with increased liver pressures elsewhere in the body. The causes for NCPH are many and include diseases that block the portal vein, such as a cancer or its spread, or a bland blood clot; rare infections, such as schistosomiasis caused by liver flukes, in which the eggs of the parasite cause intense inflammation and scarring around the small branches of the portal vein; genetic or congenital disorders of the liver such as congenital hepatic fibrosis, in which the liver develops a specific pattern of scarring that is not classic of cirrhosis; blocks in the veins that take blood away from the liver to the heart (hepatic veins), known as Budd–Chiari syndrome, named after the physicians who discovered it; heavy metal poisoning, such as chronic arsenic toxicity (the hepatoportal sclerosis type previously discussed in the prologue); disorders associated with increased blood clotting, also called prothrombotic states; and rarely, when no cause can be identified, a condition called idiopathic NCPH (commonly seen in

Western populations) or non-cirrhotic portal fibrosis (mostly from the Asian subcontinent).

Sridhar had portal hypertension, and the large shunt inside his abdomen was ferrying large volumes of non-detoxified blood rich in ammonia and other waste substances away from his liver, directly into the system and across to the brain, which was leading to brain dysfunction in the absence of advanced cirrhosis.

But what was the cause of NCPH?

Sridhar did not have a family history of liver disease or associated disorders of aggressive blood clots. His siblings were all healthy and not on medications. Even Sridhar himself had been healthy until the diagnosis of hepatic encephalopathy close to eight months earlier. Advanced-level investigations, including tests for potential unknown exposure and chronic toxicity due to arsenic, were sent out. A comprehensive genetic panel test to identify conditions associated with liver disease and high risk of clotting disorders was also sent for investigation.

Everything came back negative. Once Sridhar was well and aware of the situation, we decided to revisit his clinical history, since nothing in the tests we had sent out came back contributory. After almost an hour into questioning, Sridhar and his wife denied answers to most of our questions about his health (both factual and leading) and we were left without a cause for his portal hypertension, as Sridhar was, in all likelihood, a very healthy person who had suddenly developed an unexplainable disease.

But medical science did not ride on chances. It seeks to find the truth and evidence-based medicine is humankind's greatest ally to come closest to the truth. In the evening, Sridhar asked me to discuss his illness and further course plans. But he wanted to meet me alone in my outpatient department, and not in the inpatient room where Nayana was his bystander. As he was wheeled into my room, Sridhar talked to me about his health over the past couple of years. Sridhar and Nayana were married for three years, but they had not had children yet. They had given each other a break for a few years until they were ready to start a family. But the past couple of years had not been easy for Sridhar. Apart from the stress and anxiety of not being able to start a family and the demanding office hours, he was exhausted. A year ago, he noticed something. His left eye had turned red, painful and teary while he was visiting his hometown. He was prescribed a set of eye drops, including steroids, after which the eye symptoms resolved entirely in a couple of weeks. The doctor who treated him and the couple strongly believed it was due to a seasonal change and an allergy. It never came back.

In the past eighteen months, Sridhar had also suffered from painful, recurrent ulcers inside his mouth, but they went away in a week on a short course of painkillers and, again, on steroid paste application. This had happened more than three times.

For six months, his sex life and sexual drive had been low because the ulcers were sometimes notable at the tip of his penis, at the region known as glans. Some nights, when his wife wanted to make love, Sridhar would shy away, telling her that his mouth had ulcers when, in fact, it was the penile ulcers that he was worried she would notice. They went away in a week and returned only after many months. He thought they were stress-related.

Without waiting, while asking for the staff to return Sridhar to his room, I called the inpatient nursing staff and told them to perform a skin prick test to confirm my intuitions about what was affecting Sridhar. The skin prick test is a simple one to perform, but it can reveal a sinister disease. A small sterile needle was inserted into Sridhar's skin, over his forearm, and the area was marked. The next day, while on morning rounds, my young fellow doctor called to tell me that the result was positive. Armed with the new set of clinical symptoms Sridhar had provided, the test result seemed bittersweet. Sweet because we had a diagnosis, bitter because it was not a good one.

Approximately 2,500 years earlier, Hippocrates described a disease among people in Asia Minor, the region between the Black Sea, Aegean Sea and the Mediterranean Sea—currently known as Anatolia, the peninsula of land that today constitutes the Asian portion of Turkey.

In his description, he mentioned patients who developed painful oral ulcerations (also called aphthous ulcers), a similar affliction over the genital parts and painful watering of the eyes, which relapsed and recurred and was chronic. Centuries later, Adamantiades, a modern-day Greek physician, reported the disease in medical literature. Six years after that, in 1937, a Turkish physician and skin specialist, Hulusi Behçet, reported the same disease entity with further clarity and a set of clinically relevant diagnostic criteria, after which the disease came to be known by his name. Behçet's disease is characterized by the mandatory presence of recurrent oral ulcers, plus two of either recurrent genital ulcerations, eye disorders (called uveitis, in which the anterior or posterior part of the eyeball or blood vessels in the retina are inflamed), various types of skin lesions (commonly the severe skin condition erythema nodosum) or a positive pathergy test—also known as the skin prick test.

In Sridhar, the skin prick test was positive, meaning that a small red raised nodule with severe inflammation had developed at the site of the sterile needle prick, demonstrating the hyperactivity of his immune system. With more than three clinical criteria met, Sridhar was diagnosed with Behçet's disease, and portal hypertension in the absence of liver disease was, in all likelihood, secondary to the inflammation of the blood vessels (vasculitis) notable in Behçet's disease. The disease is seldom seen among those in Western countries, and the geographical distribution of this disease, encountered mainly in countries spanning the Mediterranean basin and the Far East, also led to it being called the Silk Road disease. The disease is associated with a heritable risk factor involving genes of the HLA-B*51 region on the chromosomes. It is explained by the earlier demographic movements across Asia and the Beringia Landmass (the Beringia Straits) some 10,000 to 30,000 years ago.

We were now closest to the truth but had not reached the summit yet. Since Behçet's disease was not described in the type of NCPH Sridhar had, we were unsure about this association. In medical literature, the most reported liver involvement in Behçet's disease was a block in the hepatic veins (also called Budd–Chiari syndrome), which had a different clinical presentation. However, in Sridhar, the hepatic veins were normal after CT imaging. To identify the genuine liver involvement, I discussed with Sridhar the need for a liver biopsy to directly see everything happening to his liver, and he agreed. The biopsy was done the next day as the pathologist processed the specimen in record time so we could review it together.

In the pathology department, I looked at the images with awe, as they were projected from the microscope onto a screen by my pathologist, and we identified a decades-old foe of the liver that had been hiding in plain sight.

In 1953, Dr S. Ranström of the Sahlgrenska Hospital, Gothenburg, Sweden, identified a peculiar finding in the liver of a person suffering from a strange complication of rheumatoid arthritis. He had a massive spleen, and his white blood cell counts were very low (neutropenia), a condition called Felty's syndrome. At the time, unable to explain the small nodules that completely replaced the liver in the absence of scar tissue development, Ranström termed the condition 'miliary liver adenomatosis' and left it at that. Six years later, Paul E. Steiner, from the University of Chicago, found a similar patient with multiple liver nodules replacing normal liver structure without any evidence for the scarring that is usually seen with cirrhosis. He called this condition nodular regenerative hyperplasia, or NRH.

As years went by, many clinical pathologists started identifying this strange disease associated with a host of other conditions, ranging from autoimmune disorders to vasculitis syndromes, notably characterized by inflammation of the blood vessels in various organ systems, including the liver. The big revelation came in 1990, when the brilliant pathologist Ian Wanless of Toronto Western Hospital, Canada, looked at the livers of 2,500 people with a cirrhosis diagnosis who had died from various illnesses. He found that around 3 per cent of these patients did not have cirrhosis, but NRH mimicked cirrhosis. However, unlike in cirrhosis, the liver nodules were not separated by scar tissue or fibrosis. The NRH was suggested to be the consequence of alterations in blood flow within the liver, mediated by immune-related damage or blood vessel inflammation.

Looking at the screen, I could see the history of medicine flash before my eyes. The presence of scarring and nodules would have been a diagnosis of classic cirrhosis. However, in Sridhar's case, there was no scarring around the nodules in the liver biopsy, which confirmed the diagnosis of the NRH type of NCPH, which was associated with Behçet's disease. Ours was not the first case. In 1992, a group of doctors diagnosed a patient with NRH associated with Behçet's disease after his death, via a post-mortem liver biopsy. We had diagnosed the same in a living person for the first time.

We published Sridhar's clinical report shortly after that as the second case of Behçet's disease with NRH of the liver, presenting with features of portal-hypertension-related brain dysfunction, and the first living patient with this rare but dreadful condition. As part of the treatment for Behçet's disease, Sridhar was started on immunosuppression drugs and a special drug called Colchicine—which effectively reduced the severity and recurrence of oral and genital ulcers—along with treatments aimed at lowering ammonia in the body and for portal hypertension. After a ten-day roller-coaster ride of hospital events, Sridhar was ultimately discharged. A man who came with memory loss and unintelligible muttering, then lay on a hospital bed with a diagnosis of cirrhosis, was sent home walking, fully rehabilitated, with a diagnosis known only in one other person who had not survived to tell the tale. Sridhar's case taught us something valuable and useful. In clinical medicine, we can never leave anything to chance. There is an explanation, a reason, and it remains hidden inside questions the physician, out of curiosity and a thirst for reason, repeatedly asks the patient—waiting for the right question at the right time, and never in the many investigational reports printed on paper.

~

Meanwhile, Harish was holding on with the extraordinary support he was receiving. The plasma exchange was in full swing, but the clinical improvement dragged. Even though he was not crashing on the ventilator, the lack of improvement worried us. It was distressing because the young man was not getting down-staged from his ACLF grade, even with the best supportive care. Published literature and the multitude of experiences of physicians caring for critically ill cirrhosis patients were all pointing towards one outcome for Harish.

Death.

When patients with ACLF remained in Grade 3 even after the best of organ support efforts, the chances of survival were almost zero. The risk of liver transplantation in this scenario far outweighed its realistic benefits. One day passed, then another, and Harish remained the same, holding on to his dear life while we supported him as he slept on the ventilator, dreaming of the unknown.

A critically ill cirrhosis patient in multiple organ failure is a situation where the role of medical science ends and the act of humanism begins. It is the time when doctors hang up their white coats and start putting themselves in the shoes of their patients' families. Treatment takes a back seat, and comfort care takes the wheel. It calls for a delicate balance in the context of thoughtful and purposeful next steps from the physician who now has the knowledge and the heartbreaking realization that the patient would depart soon. Here, comforting the patient is easy. The ventilator, the sedatives, the relaxants and the unconditional nursing care ensure it. But the real spotlight is about taking care of the family. Overnight, I contemplated how I would break the devastating news to Nalini.

I have a terrible habit. I know it is not healthy, and I must stop doing it at some point for the sake of my health and for my family. I perform a self-stress test many times, especially when my patients are critically ill. I project their situation into mine. I imagine that if I was critically sick and, on a ventilator, how a routine day would be for my wife and children. How much would that break them into a million little pieces? What would they do if I was suddenly not around? Then, to bring me to an extreme form of realization of what my patients go through, I change roles. I imagine my wife on the ventilator, critically ill and without an outcome on the horizon. Every day, a puzzle, every minute more anxious than the previous one. Me and my children alone. How would our lives be? How much would I cry? How long could I cry? How many tears shed would justify me being in that terrifying situation? What would I do?

Then I change roles again to lose one of my children, which gets me in knots around my heart every time. I never complete that role-play. It crushes me, chokes me, and I start feeling numb. Because I know we do not live forever in an unknown future, and sickness will get to us one day. When the heartache gets close enough to kill me and the pain becomes unbearable, I slide away from that imagination into reality. I take a deep breath, thankful for everything and everyone around me. I was now more aware of what Nalini was going through, and I was ready to ferry her into a world where comfort took over treatment and I became human, not a doctor.

On my way out from the morning rounds, I met Nalini outside the ICU. I took her inside an empty counselling room, which I suddenly realized was eerily silent. Then I told her calmly that Harish was going to die.

'But we do not have children,' she told me, teary-eyed. 'It will be like he never existed.'

Then came part of the response that I never expected. It did not take shape from grief or sadness. It was a response that genuinely came to be from fear. Fear of loss. Of loneliness. We all fear that. A day when we will have to face the loss of a father, mother, brother or sister, a husband, wife, daughter or son. Our sadness is only a veil for the fear. We are not truly sad; we do not grieve. We change into scared little children who have lost their parents, our adulthood compressed into our foetal selves, looking to find a way home. Nalini seemed lost.

'There would never be a part of him with me,' she told me. 'Please, doctor, can you arrange to retrieve his sperm for me to have his child?'

This was a strange response. All my life, when I gave death counselling to patients' families, I expected specific reactions to which I had comforting responses. Some got angry—losing clutches at the last straw, having nothing to hold on to and frustrated that the prognosis did not improve. Others sobbed persistently until I left the frame. The majority kept silent, their eyes brimming with tears, with occasional gulps that eased their palpable heartache. But Nalini's response caught me off-guard. Chaos broke out. Harish's parents wanted him to fade into peace in his induced sleep; they did not want any of that journey to be violated. But Nalini slipped into a passion-filled delirium that could only be reversed if she had something from Harish to hold on and look forward to. Harish suffered from alcohol use disorder; his body was replete with infection, and almost all his organs had failed. In a state of extreme shock, the heart pumped blood under force from medications that made it beat out of exhaustion and barely perfused his organs.

The Canopic Jar of Imset

In ancient Egypt, when people died, their bodies were preserved for the afterlife by mummification. The organs were stored in pottery or jars carved from limestone. All the organs did not go into a single jar. Each had its place, a sanctuary. There were four: one each for the stomach, the intestines, the lungs and the liver. Since the heart was considered the seat of the soul, it was left inside the mummified body. Each organ was guarded by one of the four sons of Horus, who were, in turn, protected by their companion goddesses. The lungs were placed inside the jar shaped like the baboon-headed god, Hapi; the jackal-headed god Duamutef's jar contained the stomach; and the falcon-headed god Qebehsenuef's jar contained the intestines. The only jar in human shape, which represented Imset, the human-headed god, contained the liver.

In the Galenic medicine of Greece, the heart was thought to give 'emotions' and the liver 'passion'. The liver was also considered the origin of blood and became the human life's epicentre. The liver descriptor term is 'hepar', of Greek origin, which arises from the word 'hedoné', meaning 'pleasure.' The initial belief was that the liver housed human desire, and because it was warm, soft and moist, it was associated with love. Because love was 'fiery', and the yellow bile was bright and plenty in the liver, this mysterious organ was considered the seat of fire. The English term 'liver' is derived from the Anglo-Saxon word 'lifere', which means 'to live'. The liver was once romanticized, and it was woefully apt that the significantly failing romanticism was tearing Nalini and Harish apart.

The ICU doctors, hospital administrators, institutional ethics committee senior members and the regional organ retrieval coordinator were all called upon to respond to the query regarding fulfilling Nalini's strange request. They agreed that if two persons from the immediate family (including Nalini) were to consent, they would go ahead and retrieve Harish's sperm for preservation. Through a procedure called the testicular sperm aspiration (TESA, in which a needle is inserted into the testes and sperm are gently sucked into a syringe) or testicular sperm extraction (TESE, in which minute cuts are placed over the testes visualized under a microscope and sperm are retrieved) the doctors were ready to fulfil Nalini's odd but loving request. But Harish's father would not consent. Since Nalini and Harish did not have children and Nalini was still young enough for a second marriage, the rationally thinking man concluded that it would be selfish of them to allow 'excess baggage' into Nalini's new life.

She would have to move on, and this could not be, under any circumstance, an obstacle to her sailing into an unknown but more hopeful future. Harish would be gone. They knew it because I confirmed it. He would remain a perfect son in their memories and a loving past in Nalini's. Time would move them into a new phase, in which everything in the past would gladden their hearts occasionally, as humans have an uncanny penchant for remembering things that made them mournfully happy.

We moved Harish into a special cabin in a corner of the ICU, away from the hustle and bustle of other patients who still had a chance at life.

In that incandescently lit cabin, Harish's mother, father and Nalini could take turns spending final moments with him as he prepared for a one-way ticket journey away from them.

During my evening rounds, I saw Nalini, her head rested partly on Harish's pillow, her hands across his chest, moving in rhythm with the oxygen that was being pumped into his chest by the mechanical ventilator. I did not go in. My presence in there as a doctor was futile. My presence there as another human being would have been an inconvenience to the flow of bittersweet thoughts Nalini was creating in her mind. I looked at the corner cabin one last time as I left the ICU.

Late at night, as I was sitting at the computer, training my mind to forget exhaustion, and trying hard to focus on completing research data analysis for recently performed clinical trials in my unit, I received a few messages on my phone from the on-call duty doctor in the ICU. A few minutes after midnight, Harish had passed away, silently but comfortably into the void, surrounded by his parents. Nalini never entered the cabin later that night to witness Harish's motionless body, off the ventilator and without the lines. In her palpable imagination, on her hands, his chest was still moving, his heart was still beating and the flow of his bittersweet thoughts remained undisturbed.

I remembered Juniper—how she died alone, surrounded by strangers. I thought of the first time I held her, full of life and hope, and the last time, holding her lifeless body. There was a journey in between, but in the end, only that final moment mattered—being there when it counted.

Too often, I saw people die without their loved ones—parents without children, children without parents, spouses saying goodbye into silence, siblings passing without a hand to hold. Life, more often unfair, sometimes denied even the simplest dignities. Juniper's incomplete goodbye haunted me, a quiet penance that now drives me to ensure others don't leave this world alone, like with Harish and his family. Sometimes, being a doctor means more than healing; it means guiding, comforting ... or simply being there.

In those final moments, there is no time for anything but presence. When someone drifts into that in-between space—neither here nor gone—what matters most is not medicine or machines, but memories, connection and the precious moments spent together.

Nalini lost Harish. I lost a young man to a monstrous disease. I lost weeks of sleep and appetite, trying to help them be together, fighting against all odds. But they were together in that memorably bittersweet eventuality. I understood it was far more important than anything medical science could offer. I understood this because I was putting myself in Nalini's and Harish's shoes on that night. I had lost my doctor self and become human. That night, I found out that being together did not mean being in an embrace in the physical context. It meant being in a loving haze during the most testing times, trapped inside cherished, aching memories.

We, the doctors and nurses, all of us human and humane, holding out for each other, had made it happen.

Because to die in love is a great thing of beauty.

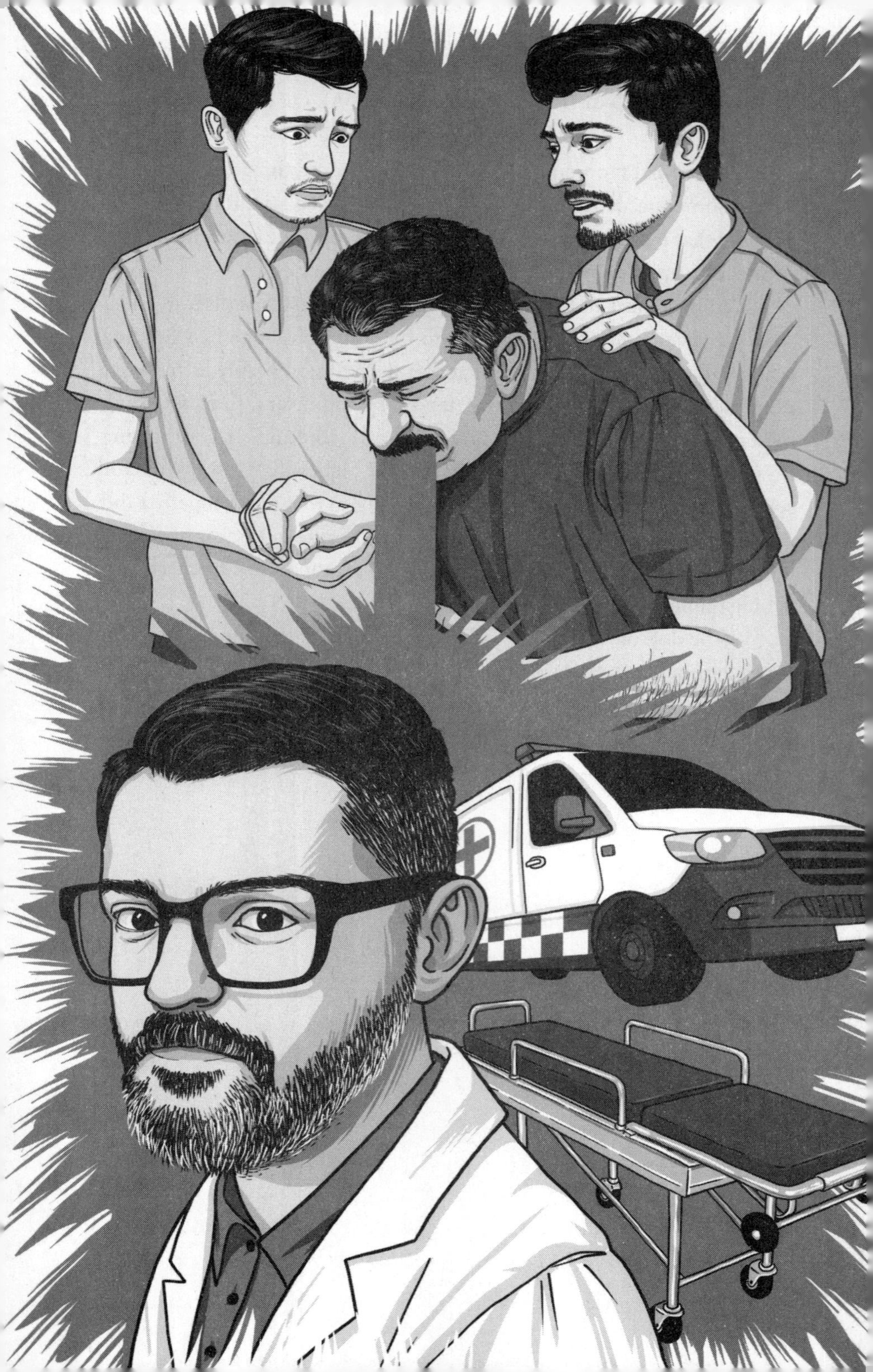

CHAPTER 3

Memento Mori

Grappling with Bleeding Complications of Liver Disease

Blood Is Thicker than Water

'Death smiles at us all; all a man can do is smile back.'
—MARCUS AURELIUS

Remember, We Must Live

WHEN FIFTY-THREE-YEAR-OLD SURESH CAME HOME LATE IN the evening, he was starving. A hard-working man, he ran a small supermarket store, starting work early and finishing after every employee left for the evening. A quick shower later, he was ready to dig into the sumptuous dinner that his wife, Nivya, had prepared for him. His two sons—Vimal, who was in high school, and Roshan, who was doing his bachelor's degree in electronics—also joined him. After a heavy meal and a bottle of beer, he retired early for bed.

However, early the next morning, Suresh woke up with an abdominal discomfort he had never felt before. Blaming it on the heavy meal and the beer he had had the previous night, he tossed and turned on his bed, trying to catch up on the rest of his sleep. But the gurgling sounds in his abdomen were getting worse, and he felt nauseous. Getting up from the bed, he felt dizzy. Holding on to the side table for balance, he slowly moved towards the bathroom as the abdominal cramps got stronger. Unable to hold on to the urge that was coming on, Suresh lost control over his defecation before he found himself inside the bathroom. And on the floor, he saw something he had never seen: black, tarry, sticky stools. This was not the end; the large volume of stools that Suresh defecated into the commode looked similar and sinister. He felt dizzy again and collapsed onto the floor, his T-shirt now plastered with the tarry faeces on the floor. He lost consciousness.

Nivya was in a surreal state of sleep when she heard a loud thud from the bathroom. Seeing the bathroom door partly ajar and the lights on, groggy and partly awake, she moved towards the light source. Seeing Suresh unresponsive on the floor, she was too frozen in time to act rationally. The scene where her husband was half-naked on the floor, the stench of strange-looking faeces in the air, overwhelmed her as she shouted at the top of her lungs for her sons.

When Suresh arrived at our emergency department later that morning, he was unresponsive. In hypovolemic shock—a condition in which blood or fluids drain out of the body through vomitus or diarrhoea and bleeding, leaving the heart to pump nothing—the blood pressure goes downhill and crashes. Once the heart winds down, the brain screams for two essentials that keep it going: glucose and oxygen. With oxygen deprivation, the brain shuts down; the brain cells start dying when oxygen supply is cut off beyond five minutes. From alteration in behaviour to confusion, seizures and finally loss of consciousness and coma, the brain gives way to the insult in a stepwise manner. In the human body, when the blood loss is extreme, automated processes kick in, which directly double the blood volume to the brain and away from other organs to maintain cognition. However, in severe blood loss, like in the case of Suresh, this damage-control mechanism does not work as intended.

In the emergency room, the attending doctor noticed the tarry, foul-smelling stools on Suresh and the copious amounts on his clothes. He knew that it was a symptom called melena. It is the presence of jet-black, tarry stools associated with bleeding from the upper gastrointestinal tract, from sources in the food pipe (oesophagus) to the upper small intestine (the lowest part of the section called the duodenum). The foul odour is strangely nauseating because the haemoglobin protein within the red blood cells, which carry oxygen, gets digested in the gut by acid, enzymes and intestinal bacteria. Iron supplements and foods such as beetroot, blueberries and black licorice can also darken stools, but they do not cause them to be loose and reeking anomalous like melenic stools. When washed off, the melenic stools stain the clothes and surface an intensely dark red.

Suresh was in danger. He was drifting in and out of consciousness, fighting a losing battle to stay awake. There was a danger of him aspirating his oral secretions and a high risk of blood clots in the stomach being aspirated into the lungs. The rule-book pages of emergency management in a bleeding patient losing consciousness flip through the attending physician's mind. His airway had to be secured and his breathing settled, while they pumped packed red blood cells into Suresh to get his blood pressure up and running.

In minutes, a long, curved tube went into Suresh's large airway, which led from the voice box (larynx) to the common path that opens into the lungs. The tube was secured in place, and Suresh was connected to a mechanical ventilator that would help him breathe while sedated and relaxed. The blood transfused into Suresh was not helping to increase the fluid volume enough to maintain his blood pressure. The emergency physicians started him on a group of medications called inotropes, which are drugs that help the heart muscles beat and contract with more power. This helps maintain blood pressure in the body, enough for the other organs and tissues to bathe in blood and perfuse aptly to perform their functions. Once Suresh was stabilized, the nurses, along with the emergency doctors, rolled him out to another department of hardened physicians who could take over the preservation of Suresh's life: the ICU.

As Suresh was wheeled into the medical ICU, the bag of blood hanging on the side, tubes and lines going in and out of his body, and a large machine breathing for him, the ICU doctor stepped in to check his vitals. The blood transfusion and the inotropes were keeping his blood pressure stable, but the stress of losing a large volume of blood had taken a toll on him. His kidneys were still not hurt, since the side urine bag showed adequate collection. Since he was clinically stabilized, the ICU team called in the gastroenterology physician on call to get to the heart of the matter.

An upper gastrointestinal endoscopy was the first intervention that had to be performed for two important reasons: one, to identify the source of bleeding in the gut; and two, to control the bleeding by treating that source. This was done using an oesophago-gastro duodenoscopy, or OGD procedure, in short. A flexible tube with a mini camera, light source and multiple channels was introduced into the throat and pushed into the food pipe and stomach of a sedated Suresh. What the endoscopist saw was something terrible. Large, fresh, jelly-like blood clots had filled his food pipe and stomach. Identifying the part that was bleeding was almost impossible. But he did find something valuable. Through all that bloody mess, he saw large, tortuous, bulbous structures protruding into the food pipe—some of them a deep-bluish hue, while others had angry red stripes. He now knew why Suresh had bled. He also knew every decision from that moment on had to be made quickly and purposefully. Otherwise, death was imminent for Suresh on that ventilator.

The structures that terrified the endoscopist were called varices—large, abnormal and snake-like veins that form inside the food pipe, stomach and intestines in patients with portal hypertension. Portal hypertension can be secondary to a deformed or shrunken liver, which we know as cirrhosis. It can also occur in the absence of cirrhosis, which you may recall from chapter 2, is known as NCPH. A bedside ultrasound revealed that Suresh had a shrunken liver. He had cirrhosis, and this was the first presentation of that dreadful disease—a complication called acute variceal bleeding. The doctor knew what he had to do instantly.

~

During the fifth century BCE, Hippocrates described various methods to treat bleeding haemorrhoids (commonly called piles), which are swollen veins in the anus and rectum that cause discomfort and bleeding—like varices found inside the food pipe and stomach in patients with cirrhosis. Initial attempts at treating such swollen blood vessels were crude and inhumane. The patient was held down, arms restrained by assistants, while the physician inserted red-hot surgical instruments into the anus to burn and dry out the swollen veins. This would create large wounds, which would then be taken care of using herbal dressings containing honey. However, as time passed, Hippocrates developed a process to replace this crude practice. He would manually tie woollen threads at the base of the swollen haemorrhoidal veins to cut off its blood supply, and after that, the vessel bunch would fall off. This was probably the first time a 'band-ligation' technique was described in ancient medical literature.

Dr Paul C. Blaisdell refined rubber band ligation (tying up) of haemorrhoids in 1958. However, the repeated manual ligation procedure during a single sitting was tedious. So in early 1963, James Barron invented the Barron ligator, which consisted of a haemorrhoid-grasping forceps over which a drum loaded with rubber bands was placed for repeated and easy release of bands around the base of the bleeding vessel. Before 1970, in patients with cirrhosis who bled from varices in the oesophagus and stomach, surgical management of the bleeding source was the only option. Surgeons would open the site of bleeding and cut out the bleeding part of the food pipe (called oesophagectomy) or staple the bleeding vessels, shutting them tight. Later, they would either try to remove all the abnormally engorged bleeding veins (a procedure called devascularization), ligate the veins one by one, or inject a chemical into the bleeding veins to scar and prevent them from rupturing further (a process called sclerotherapy). The latter was initially performed by Crafoord and Freckner in 1939, when they injected quinine into the bleeding varices inside the food pipe.

When rigid (and later, narrow) fibre-optic endoscopes were introduced, the requirement for opening people up to stop them from bleeding at the cost of other surgical stress-related adverse effects became obsolete, and endoscopy-guided sclerotherapy injections became the norm. Sclerotherapy injection, using a host of newly identified and neutral chemicals, became the go-to therapy when patients came in with bleeding from varices.

But, in the late 1980s, taking a hint from what Hippocrates did during ancient times, and taking a leaf out of the surgeon's lesson book on banding bleeding haemorrhoids, a group of researchers tried the band-ligation technique in the form of experiments on dogs who presented with cirrhosis or who were bleeding from varices. Dr Greg Van Stiegmann (of the department of surgery, University of Colorado Health Sciences Center, and Denver Veterans Administration Hospital in Denver, Colorado), along with his colleague, found that band ligation using an over-the-scope device, very similar to the mechanism of the Barron ligator, was effective in controlling bleeding from varices and obliterating them when bands were applied at the base of the vein while the vessel was sucked into a tubular chamber of the endoscope. After their dog experiments, the team successfully performed the first band ligation treatment of varices in humans in 1988. Endoscopic variceal band ligation (EVBL) is still the recommended first choice for the treatment and control of bleeding varices in patients with cirrhosis.

Back in the ICU, removing the scope from Suresh's insides, the endoscopist got ready to perform a decades-old procedure to save the man's life. He quickly asked his assisting technical staff to fix a band ligator device over the scope. The endoscope was reintroduced, with the bands attached to Suresh's food pipe. The erratic gushes of blood from the walls of the food pipe, from large bleeding varices hitherto unseen within a blood field, were difficult for the young endoscopist to tackle. However, with precision, focus and purposeful movement, he directed the scope towards the junction of the food pipe and the stomach, where the abnormal veins naturally originate. Blind but focused, with a soaring heart rate under absolute blood-red vision, he sucked at the bulbous structures there. In quick succession, he applied bands at their base through fast movements of the scope wheel. In a matter of seconds, he saw that the gushing had stopped, and the pale pink colour of the lining of the food pipe was now visible.

After removing the instrument, the endoscopist looked at Suresh's vitals and jotted them down in his notes for further monitoring. He found them to be adequately stable. The ICU doctors monitored Suresh's vitals like hawks, looking for unexpected changes while he slept comfortably, supported by the ventilator. But little did they know that a couple of hours later, they would face a terrifying complication that would give them palpable anxiety—that everything they had done until now would be in vain.

Remember, We Must Fight

When I received the call about Suresh, every little fundamental aspect of following protocols in an acutely bleeding patient had been followed to the T by the on-duty team. I looked at Suresh's file and his clinical history. He was a healthy man who had never been to a hospital until now, when he was fighting for his life. Acute variceal bleeding is the first presentation of complicated cirrhosis in approximately 30 per cent of patients. The most common complication of unstable cirrhosis is ascites, in which, as you may recall from earlier sections, fluid accumulates inside the abdominal cavity. The volume of blood flowing into the portal vein is 1,500 ml per minute. When the liver becomes cirrhotic, the stiffness increases, which blocks blood flow into the liver. The blood then flows away from the liver and into large, abnormal blood channels that develop in the digestive tract. When stressed, these channels burst, leading to the clinical presentation of blood vomitus or passage of black, tarry stools. Around 20 per cent of patients with variceal bleeding die within the first six weeks after the episode. Twenty per cent of those who experience variceal bleeding do not respond to the standard methods of care, such as medical and endoscopic treatments. These patients experience what is called either 'failure to control bleeding' or 'rebleeding'—the latter occurring within forty-eight hours after the first endoscopy. Any bleeding event beyond that is considered a recurrent bleed.

After Suresh's bleeding was stabilized, the next step was to ensure he did not develop an infection post bleed. Severe bacterial infections are common in patients with cirrhosis who bleed massively. Once the infection sets in, it is almost the endgame. So the ICU physicians pumped in empirical antibiotics to prevent infections.

Outside the medical ICU, two sons and a wife waited to hear a hopeful update about the head of their family. I saw them for the first time and brought them up to date first about the disease and what it could do to the human body. I told them that complications came without warning and people died without saying real goodbyes. Massive bleeding akin to what Suresh faced would kill many. But he was holding—holding on to them and not ready to let go.

An hour after I comforted the family and modified Suresh's medications, I got a frantic call from the ICU. Suresh's blood pressure was dropping. Fluid boluses and increased dosing of inotropes were not helping. He was going to crash, and a cardiac arrest was imminent. Something terrible was happening. I rushed inside the ICU and saw a bunch of nursing staff drawing blood, some suctioning fresh blood clots out of Suresh's mouth while others were pumping freshly packed red cells into his extensive intravenous neck access.

Everything was chaotic. Beautifully chaotic. Exactly how an ICU should be. Every healthcare worker had a purpose and homed in on the sickest person inside the room: my dying patient. Without instructions, they fulfilled their tasks with precise and targeted roles that spontaneously embraced their minds as they faced monstrous adversity. Every single person in that ICU was clutching at the last straws to salvage a life. I stood there with a hollow heart and racing mind, unable to process emotion, forced instead to focus on saving Suresh. In medicine, we're taught a hidden curriculum—a quiet conspiracy of silence—that trains us to suppress emotion, to disconnect just enough to function under pressure. While some become cold and clinical, I absorbed it differently—letting the grief in, storing it until there was space to mourn. But that moment wasn't now; this was the window to act. Earned through years of training, this was where purpose met pressure, where a doctor's mind must be strongest precisely when the heart feels weakest, the true test of everything we study: the fight to save a life.

~

In 1945, Dr Arthur Hendley Blakemore, at the department of surgery of Columbia New York Presbyterian Hospital, witnessed large numbers of cirrhosis patients dying of bleeding from varices. Many patients reached the hospital from peripheral centres in an exsanguinated state and died soon, before the doctors could successfully operate to control the bleeding. At the time, endoscopic techniques for the control of bleeding had not evolved yet, and a complicated and morbid surgical procedure known as 'portocaval shunt creation' was the only way to stop patients from haemorrhaging to death. However, this surgery by itself was associated with high death rates in advanced liver disease patients with uncontrolled bleeding. There had to be an interim method that arrested the bleeding and stabilized patients, buying doctors enough time to provide definitive care or perform surgery in a more conducive environment. Dr Blakemore found his idea taking shape with the help of a neurologist working at the same hospital, Dr Robert Sengstaken. In 1950, both physicians published a practice-changing paper on what came to be known as the Sengstaken–Blakemore tube, or the SB tube.

This device is a large rubber tube with two balloons, one in the middle and one at the end, which can be inflated and expansion-controlled when filled with air or water. The tube is placed in the stomach through the nose or mouth, and air or water is injected into the channel that connects to the balloon in the stomach. Once the balloon is inflated up to capacity, the tube is steadily and softly pulled out, and traction is placed. In the process, the inflated balloon rests firmly and stiffly at the junction of the food pipe and the beginning of the stomach, where the large bleeding vessels originate, effectively choking the blood flow there. If this is not effective, the long balloon in the food pipe is also inflated to compress the bleeding vessels directly. The SB tube gained popularity because it was a straightforward approach to stop bleeding from varices in cirrhosis patients who needed to be optimized before surgery and, in the current era, endoscopy. The simple 'balloon tamponade' procedure using the SB tube thus became a cornerstone of the management of varices that bleed uncontrollably.

~

I called the chief nursing staff to bring out the SB tube. In a matter of minutes, the whole process of the insertion of the tube, inflation, traction and the placement of the fixture was completed. The sizeable inflated balloon rested firmly at the junction of the food pipe and stomach, not allowing the blood to flow into the haemorrhaging vessels.

As the bleeding reduced, Suresh's blood pressure started to pick up in minutes to hours. The SB tube was doing what it was supposed to, providing the same benefit noted with its use in 1950. We had twenty-four hours before we could do something definitive for Suresh, because there was a caveat. An SB tube could not be kept for more than twenty-four hours because before the pressured placement would start eroding into the walls of the stomach and food pipe, causing damage and rupture. Now, there was only one attempt left. It was adventurous. It could kill Suresh. But it would also be his best bet at returning to a loving family waiting for him to get better. I picked up my phone and called my chief of interventional radiology.

Remember, We Must Breathe

In 1968, Dr Josef Rösch, originally from Czechoslovakia (now split into the Czech Republic and Slovakia), was invited by Dr Charles Dotter at the University of Oregon Medical School to work as a research fellow on a technique known as transjugular cholangiography—a procedure in which the bile duct inside the liver was accessed by placing a guided wire inside a vein in the neck, which was then coursed through the right side of the heart and then through the large vein that drains the liver. However, during the procedure, Rösch inadvertently punctured the portal vein. By accident, the doctors discovered that the portal vein could also be accessed by guiding a wire through the veins in the neck—a technique now known as transjugular portal access.

This was followed by various experiments on dogs, in which researchers tried accessing the portal vein through the neck vein and placed a stent between two blood vessels within the liver: the hepatic vein (that takes blood away from the liver), a naturally low-pressure system; and the portal vein (that brings blood into the liver), which develops high liver pressures within it in the presence of a shrunken, stiff and rigid liver. This procedure was called transjugular intrahepatic portosystemic shunt placement, or TIPS. When blood flow from the portal vein was diverted into the hepatic vein through an artificially placed stent, the liver pressures were reduced, and complications related to high portal vein pressure (or portal hypertension) were abolished. Early attempts at maintaining patency of the stent failed miserably, until the late 1980s and 1990s, when bare metal stents were replaced by polytetrafluoroethylene-coated ones that helped the process, avoiding early clot formation once TIPS was created.

The twenty-four-hour time limit for the SB tube was running out for Suresh. He was getting too sick to be transported to the cath lab for a TIPS procedure. The ICU doctors had to take the call, and it was as easy as apple pie. If Suresh were to remain in the ICU with the SB tube on, the chances of him dying were far greater than the high-risk shift to the cath lab for a potentially life-saving procedure. So they put their best ICU fellows on Suresh, who wheeled him directly into the interventional radiology procedure suite late in the evening. The family consented to the procedure because its risks were weighed against one dreadful outcome: an old friend, Death.

Someone once said, 'When you own your breath, nobody can steal your peace.' We decided to own Suresh's breath and not hand it over to Death, and in that adrenaline-rushed stress that skyrocketed inside our hearts and minds, we found peace for Suresh. In a matter of twenty minutes, my interventional radiology chief skilfully placed a stent between the portal vein and the hepatic vein after creating a path within the liver, in a comatose and ventilated Suresh. Like a miracle entirely conjured by humans working in tandem for one purpose—to save a life—the doctors performing the procedure saw the liver pressure drop in minutes. In real time, they watched as the large blood vessels inside Suresh's food pipe and stomach withered away under the presence of the newly introduced liver stent. The bleeding was controlled.

Now, there was this other endgame. Suresh had to wake up. The massive amount of bleeding and then the rebleeding had taken a toll on his brain, with the extensive rise in ammonia levels in his body. I pumped up the medical management to wash out all that ammonia. At the same time, the ICU doctors slowly and steadily started to reduce Suresh's medical sedation, giving him a chance to wake up spontaneously.

Two days passed, and Suresh was not showing any signs of waking up, even after complete cessation of all sedation. Researchers and philosophers have long contended the quantitative presence of an unconscious mind. For neuroscientists, the unconscious mind is a sanctuary where the brain processes information outside awareness. Studies and large-scale analysis suggest strong evidence that some patients diagnosed as being in a 'vegetative state' can hear and understand what is being said in their environment. Interviews with previously unconscious patients and methods to measure brain activity have shed light on the fact that awareness can be detected in patients 'perceived' to be unconscious. Every day during evening rounds, I would see Suresh's sons and wife take turns whispering soft little things into his ears during visiting hours. They did this for two whole days without breaks and, sometimes, asked me special permission to speak to their father outside of visiting hours.

'He can hear us,' they would always tell me.

Can he? I always wondered. He was not brain-dead. His brain activity measures were classic signs of a liver coma, and there was no seizure activity. He was asleep, and no one could ever know what was going through his mind and all that he saw in that surreal state.

When a person fails to respond with an action to a verbal command—that requires hearing, understanding and engagement in specific brain regions that fire coordination activity, and ultimately help move particular muscle groups to complete the task—we term them 'unresponsive'. But they are not *wholly* unresponsive. Studies have shown that a condition called 'covert cognition' exists among unconscious patients in the ICU. In this state, brain activity lights up meaningfully but without the final expected action. These patients are alive and well, and can comprehend, but they are neither here nor there. Stuck in limbo, they wade through unchartered memories to finally clutch at the ones they recognize, and then rise like a balloon, free and floating, towards the light.

In the many critically ill patients I have cared for, I knew which ones would go away, come what may. If a lousy outcome were waiting to happen, given time, nothing could stop that. No prayers, no hope, no medical science or the doctor's experience or wisdom—none of it mattered. There are objective clinical scores in the medical literature that help physicians identify inevitable death among critically ill cirrhosis patients. Every score I applied to Suresh returned with a resounding hope that he would rise from the chaos in an orderly fashion. For me, the assumption of a God—a higher power that would mediate to deviate bad happenings from the chaotic good—lay in those clinical scores, and so we waited. We waited without losing hope, but refrained from giving out promises that everything was going to be okay because, on the ground, it was just me and my team of immensely aggressive physicians, always looking to pick a fight with Death. We were fighting for Suresh and his family.

Remember, We Must Die

Then, on the third day, the ICU bed nurse found Suresh's eyes fluttering and little fingers moving, and she called out to the doctor on call. Slowly, steadily and consistently, when the doctor pressed over Suresh's chest, on his sternal bone, an area of intense pain perception, he winced—a sign of awakening. Twelve hours later, Suresh's eyes were wide open but confused. Confused to see a tube going inside his mouth and into his throat, which was stopping him from speaking. But his eyes told us a lot. The ICU physician softly and slowly told Suresh that he was on a ventilator and that he had been sleeping for a long time. If he remained calm, breathed slowly and steadily, and cooperated with them, they would remove the tube as early as possible. To comfort him, they brought in Vimal, Roshan and Nivya. Even though they were all apart and standing around him, I imagined them in a tight hug, and I felt it.

Home was only a few days away. Suresh was doing well. His breathing was steady but slightly laboured, which was expected, and his oxygen levels were maintained with minimal supplementation. I spoke with the critical unit doctors, held Vimal's and Roshan's hands tight, and then retired to my outpatient department to see new patients.

In the evening, I got a call from the ICU. They were ready to remove the ventilator support from Suresh, as he was cooperating. But an X-ray of the chest done earlier that day showed a small patch on his right lung. It looked like evolving pneumonia had probably developed because Suresh had been on the ventilator for a while and had initially micro-aspirated blood when he had that massive bleed. But the pneumonia appeared to be under control, as he had no systemic symptoms. So they weaned Suresh off the ventilator, put him on supplemental oxygen and started him on speech rehabilitation and chest physiotherapy. A day later, Suresh was out of the ICU and in a single room with his family. To cover for potential ventilator-acquired pneumonia, and with the development of a new patch in the lung on his X-ray, antibiotics were upgraded before he was shifted out. Suresh did well and was scheduled for discharge over the weekend.

~

Room number A312, on the third floor. During my days on clinical rounds, I would see three chairs instead of the routine two, and all three around the bed, never near the table and one at the foot end of the bed. The room had a typical aroma—of humans and used sheets, and of rice and curries that the family enjoyed while Suresh was being rehabilitated. Every day, my rounds team would see Suresh and provide me feedback on his progress. Every day, Nivya, Vimal or Roshan would meet me in the outpatient department to discuss the continued need for follow-up care and future surveillance. Every day felt like it usually did, a routine we all drove through without any worries. Patients with cirrhosis are unpredictable. Suresh had come in on the fifth stage of cirrhosis, which involved liver failure and brain dysfunction precipitated by a bleed. We had dragged his disease stage down to two through the marvel of medical science, human compassion, sacrifice and hoping against all odds.

On the third day of rehabilitation in the room, Suresh started showing signs of an infection. Early on, the fever came in low and infrequent, but by night, it had risen to 40°C (104°F), with chills and rigors. The on-call doctor saw him at night and advised intravenous paracetamol to bring the fever down and sent blood cultures to look for any bacterial growth we could target. By morning, the fever had settled, but Suresh had become delirious, unable to identify his family members and had failed to consume breakfast. Junior doctors from my team who rushed in for an early round that morning called me to inform me that Suresh would require to be shifted back to the medical ICU for better and continued monitoring. He was not looking well. In front of a bewildered family, a confused and muttering Suresh on the bed trolley was once again wheeled into the ICU, with the same team that had fought hard to place him out of their care.

Sepsis. This condition, when an infection overwhelms the body so much that organ failures ensue, is commonly encountered in advanced liver disease patients, especially after episodes of variceal bleeding. This is one of the primary reasons why bleeding cirrhosis patients are started on an antibiotic to ward off potentially lethal infections that may kill them eventually. We had followed everything by the book and beyond while caring for a bleeding Suresh, but a sepsis event was inevitable.

However, we were not done yet.

Suresh was back in the woods. We pumped into him some of the most potent antibiotics discovered by humankind to eclipse the bacterial surge inside him. But it was not working the way we wanted it to. The fevers persisted, and the brain failure was progressing. Suresh was going into a coma, like the first time, but only this time, the reasons for it were not easy to handle. He was not bleeding; the TIPS had taken care of that. Over the next twenty-four hours, Suresh was in and out of consciousness but maintained his oxygen levels. A repeat X-ray revealed that the patch was slightly more prominent than before. However, the blood cultures sent thirty-six hours earlier grew something we had not expected and covered for—a terrifying bacterium, immensely resilient to treatment, a multi-drug-resistant strain that would be the stuff of nightmares: *Pseudomonas aeruginosa*. The demonic microbe had started as a focal area of pneumonia inside Suresh's right lung and spread to his bloodstream, knocking off his organs one by one as it ravaged his body. And the antibiotics we were pumping into him were proving to be futile.

By late evening, Suresh was non-responsive and his oxygen levels started to fall. He needed the mechanical ventilator again—to sustain life and to begin a second battle to go back home. But this time, it was different. When I spoke to Nivya and the sons, the aura had changed. There was no hope. They spoke less and less; they often just heard me but did not react. It was morose. A cloud of melancholy suddenly replaced the hopefulness we had so challengingly created out of chaos.

The money had run out. They were left high and dry from a financial point of view. They could not afford another ventilator event because it would mean that they would have to pawn whatever was left of the house and the small property, and even sell the business to keep Suresh alive—a scenario that was not guaranteed even with the most aggressive medical measures. After all, this was not a bleed we were dealing with but a foe far more powerful and potentially unstoppable. I asked them to give me forty-eight hours to work on Suresh, because the team had fought hard to get them all under one meaningful roof. Nivya did not meet me from then on, and I always dealt with either Vimal or Roshan regarding decisions. It seemed like she had made up her mind and wanted me to make up mine—one that did not involve the complete annihilation of their family's future. I realized I was fighting a battle without soldiers. I was giving hope but not weapons. Hope does not win wars; actions do. I did not have anything actionable, only motivation and strong words. Vimal and Roshan were studying, but their studies were getting hampered. If they did continue with my plan of another round at salvaging Suresh, it would mean that the funds allocated for their education would thin out, and their futures would be impacted.

Back home—while having a bath, during dinner, while going to sleep, and in my sleep—I had to convince myself to do the most challenging thing: to let go of a patient, even though I wanted to continue my fight for them. I was trying to teach myself to understand that life was not about one person but everyone around the person too. In making negative or positive decisions, one had to take the path of least resistance, which may lead to a better one later in life but was still burdened with loss and pain.

Suresh's family could not decide because I was their obstacle. I was still holding on when they had already loosened their grip. My focus on salvaging a potentially dying patient was making their lives difficult.

Suresh's death would tear them apart, but they would learn to grow around it because they had built memories, strong ones, which featured them engaging as a single unit in vigorous combat against not one but multiple challenges. They had used impossible and unimaginable effort and all their resources to save their numero uno family member.

And I was part of it too.

The next day, I witnessed Nivya signing off documents that contained end-of-life care decisions. She signed off on the page that mentioned the dreadful letters 'DNR' (Do Not Resuscitate), which meant that Suresh would not be provided life-saving measures when he sank into multiple organ failure and developed a cardiac arrest. I saw that Nivya was relieved, but she had already become the shell of the person she once was. Vimal and Roshan were around her, and the three walked into their allotted room, waiting for the inevitable.

No matter who we are or what we do, the one universal truth is that we all die. Marcus Aurelius wrote, 'You could leave life right now. Let that determine what you do and say and think.' This echoes the ancient Roman tradition where, even in the height of a general's victory parade, a slave would whisper 'memento mori'—remember, you must die. It was a sobering reminder that even in our greatest triumphs, we remain mortal, and all glory fades in the face of death. True to Marcus Aurelius's reminder, I chose my words carefully as I met with Nivya, Vimal and Roshan while on my rounds.

I told them, 'I am sorry.'

And I saw their faces crushing under the burden of loss and the fact that even I had let go.

Late that night, Suresh developed a fatal cardiac arrest. The doctors and the nurses who cared for him through his first battle watched as he flatlined. A strong heart was dying out with silent cries. The ICU doctor on call jotted down his time of death and sent me a message. I was preparing for my sleep after putting down a whole lot of burden that I carried around throughout the day at the hospital. And then this message caught my eye.

There is a strange feeling when your mind is tired and your patient dies after a tough battle. An indescribable feeling. Momentarily, and in parallel, you feel both heavy like a boulder and as light as a feather, and a flurry of aches of low and high intensity rush into your chest. You experience love and hate for being a doctor. Hate because a victory remained unsatisfied, and love thinking of that glorious fight and the near triumph that brought together strangers in the sanctuary of clinical medicine.

Clinical medicine is the hill I am willing to die on.

The next day, during clinical rounds on the third floor, I saw that room number A312 was vacant. The family had signed the final papers, cleared their dues and taken Suresh's body for cremation. The last time I saw Suresh was when he was breathless, in and out of consciousness in the ICU, unable to identify me. During his last days, Suresh could not identify me or his family as he blacked out into a second coma.

I peeped into the room and saw fresh sheets on the bed. The chairs were arranged around the table, not near the bed or at the foot end. I saw two chairs and not the usual three, which I was happily adjusted to seeing over the preceding few weeks. I smelled the fresh room deodorant—the scent of humans and used sheets had ceased to exist. I spent a few minutes at the doorstep before moving to the next room, where a stable patient was waiting to be discharged.

The senior floor nurse told me, 'A new patient is being shifted from the emergency to room number A312, and he is going to be under you, sir, in hepatology.'

Are there no other rooms for them to admit a new patient under me? I thought. I wanted a break from this room.

'Oh, I was not informed about a new patient,' I told her.

'He seems stable, and your team member has already seen and advised evaluation and baseline management measures. You could probably see the patient and speak with the family once they settle in.'

'Okay, I'll follow up on the new admission,' I told her.

Another patient and his family would distract me from Suresh and his family in minutes. Patients come and go, the sheets are changed and the chairs are rearranged. But memories remain, and I will keep them as sweet scars in a corner of my heart, which I wear on my sleeve.

Look behind.

Remember, we are all mortal.

Remember, we must all die.

But be kind, fight for and live this day because tomorrow may never come.

Because, as Rumi said, 'The wound is the place where the light enters you.'

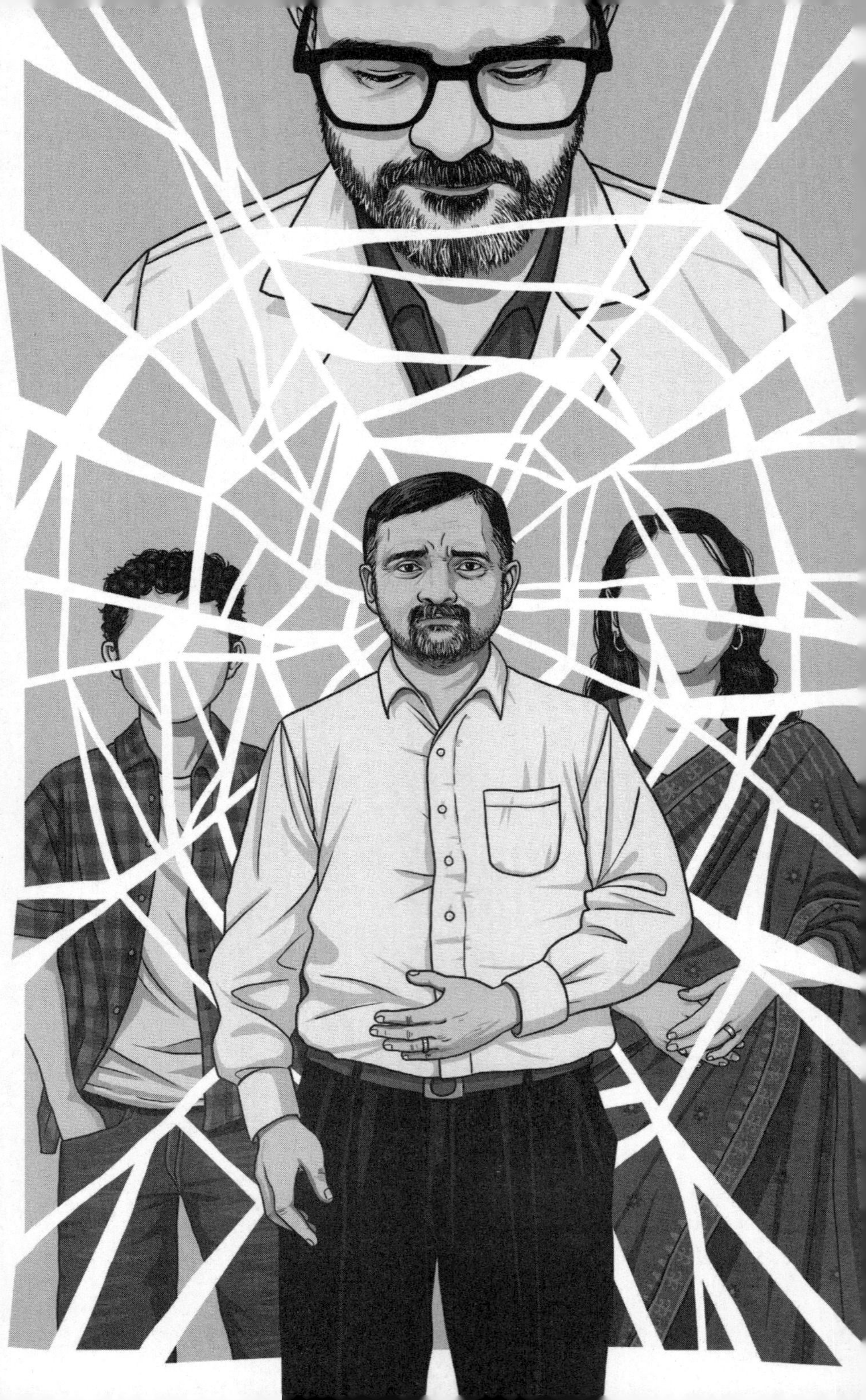

CHAPTER 4

Visceral and Cerebral

The Brain in Liver Disease

Drifting from the Shore

'No one is so brave that he is not disturbed by something unexpected.'
—Julius Caesar

The Abusive Patient and the Quiet One

What if, one day, you suddenly ceased to recognize your family?

What if, one day, you woke up and realized that the world you have known so far was not the same anymore?

As a doctor, have you ever taken care of a patient with liver disease and found yourself lost?

Cirrhosis is unforgiving.

It moves at its own pace.

Without an iota of concern or regard for challenging your existence.

It was a typical day at the hospital. I planned to meet with my follow-up patients and educate newly registered patients about the complexities of various liver diseases and their management. I had a detailed picture of how that day would unfold. Then I received an unexpected call as I was heading to the outpatient department. I needed to see and admit a patient who was referred to me. The patient's condition had the emergency physician on pins and needles. On a day that could only be described as clichéd, I veered off my course towards the outpatient services and dashed to the emergency room, where I found a young man waiting by his father, who was lying still on the bed.

'What is your father's name?' I asked Ravi, who appeared embarrassed, his hands trembling as he gazed at his father lying on the green-sheeted emergency ward bed.

Hiding his guilt but not his disdain, he answered, 'Ramesh … This has never happened before. My father defecated in front of us, in front of my cousins, and on the dining room table.'

He appeared to be in disbelief at the pace of events.

'And what did you do?' I asked Ravi.

'I made an effort to bring him down, and then …' Ravi distanced himself from the conversation, took a little pause and then, after clumsily gathering himself, said, 'He called me a son of a bitch.'

He continued as his lips quivered and contorted. He fought back the tears coming to his eyes.

~

Ramesh, a teetotaller with diabetes that was well-controlled with medication, was at his nephew's house two days prior for a birthday celebration.

He ate a full, meaty meal for dinner, stayed up late and woke up early in the morning all drowsy and muttering. He recognized his wife but had forgotten her name, and his speech was garbled. After noticing this, his wife immediately used their glucometer—a portable, point-of-care blood glucose monitoring gadget they always carried—to check his blood sugar. Hypoglycaemia, or low blood sugar, causes several clinical symptoms, including slurring of speech, anxiety, abnormal behaviour, increased sweating, tremors, shakiness and, in severe cases, seizures and coma. Ramesh's fasting glucose level, however, was normal.

Ramesh dragged himself out of bed and went to the dining room, where Ravi and other family members chatted. Ravi thought his father was acting strangely and appeared to be lost. Ramesh got up on the chair and onto the dining table before anyone could step in. He then proceeded to urinate and defecate on the table in front of every terrified individual in that room. After that, Ramesh began verbally insulting everyone who attempted to assist or remove him from the table, including his son, as his wife looked on in shock. Ramesh was eventually forced into a car and hurriedly taken to a local clinic, but only with tremendous difficulty and after heroic efforts by family members.

Did he have a stroke, perhaps? The frightened family pondered this possibility.

Ramesh was quickly examined at a local clinic. The emergency physician determined that he was exhibiting symptoms (what the patient or family complained of at presentation) and signs (what the clinician sees and feels during a clinical examination) of a stroke.

Cerebrovascular accidents, also known as strokes, occur when blood flow is cut off to a portion of the brain because of a clot (medically referred to as an ischemic stroke) or when a blood vessel bursts and bleeds into the brain matter (a haemorrhagic stroke). These events can result in behavioural changes, seizures, paralysis or sensory loss. Initially, a CT scan of the brain is used to assess this without the infusion of contrast dye. This scan result was normal for Ramesh. Blood tests received from the emergency lab were non-contributory, as were measurements of blood sugar and electrolyte levels of sodium, potassium and magnesium—alterations that might result in tremors, paralysis or abnormal behaviour.

Unexpectedly, and to the surprise of the emergency attending physician, the blood ammonia result was relatively high. The radiologist who performed the ultrasound imaging of Ramesh's abdomen called in to let them know that the liver was coarse, small and had uneven borders, which were indicators of cirrhosis or chronic liver disease. Ramesh's mental state was shifting between periods of confusion and agitation, and he was showing signs of slipping into a liver coma due to high ammonia in the blood (also known as hyperammonemia), necessitating urgent ICU care. With this new information, he was hastily referred to our unit.

Ramesh, now diagnosed with cirrhosis, was going through an ailment known as hepatic encephalopathy, which we've discussed previously as well.

~

As mentioned earlier, over 2,400 years ago, Hippocrates first linked brain dysfunction to liver disease, describing how (the now obsolete theory of) imbalances in the four bodily humours—particularly yellow bile which was believed to cause jaundice and severe irritability. This was an early account of what we now recognize as hepatic encephalopathy. Roman physicians like Celsus and Galen noted similar behavioural changes in jaundiced patients, though the true cause remained uncertain. Centuries later, Shakespeare's Sir Andrew Aguecheek, a heavy drinker in *Twelfth Night,* hinted at diet-induced cognitive decline, later inspiring the term 'Aguecheek's disease' for liver-related brain dysfunction. In the eighteenth century, Giovanni Morgagni documented its progressive stages in an alcoholic nobleman with cirrhosis, while Parisian neurologist Émile Parmentier observed meat intolerance in such patients—offering early clinical insight into the liver–brain connection.

But why were persons with chronic liver disease developing episodic features of brain failure? That question was answered in 1877 when Nikolai Vladimirovitch Eck, a Russian military surgeon, documented his experiments on eight dogs. Using a surgical technique, he connected the liver's main blood supply (called the portal vein, as we know) to the main blood vessel that drains blood from the abdomen and lower limbs (called the inferior vena cava), thereby diverting the blood flow within the liver directly into the systemic (or whole body) circulation. By doing so, he found that symptoms of 'nervousness' developed in the animals without warning, changing their behaviour.

Tame, obedient dogs became violent and vicious, moving back and forth inside the cage and chewing on items in their vicinity. Excitation was punctuated by periods of depression that progressed to deep coma and death in some. By the end of the follow-up, Eck had lost seven of his dogs this way, and the only surviving dog later ran out of the lab, its fate unknown. Eck could not describe the reasons for these findings at the time.

In 1893, Martin John Hahn at the Institut für experimentelle Medizin, St. Petersburg, Russia, recreated Eck's experiments on a new set of dogs. After the surgery, when the dogs were served meat, the ones who ran towards the meat and ate contently paid a considerable price—all of them developed a severe attack of brain dysfunction closely followed by death.

Interestingly, in Hahn's experiment, the dogs that feasted on bread, milk or oatmeal did not develop brain failure. When the meat was stopped in the dogs that developed acute behavioural changes, they returned to normal. Hahn and his colleagues called this phenomenon meat poisoning, or encephalitis (brain infection) due to meat intoxication, because the brain tissue of the dead dogs showed severe inflammation and swelling at necropsy (pet autopsy).

The Italian zoologist and doctor Filippo De Filippi hypothesized that since only meat-based diets precipitated brain failure in dogs, the liver in these dogs after the surgery could not handle high amounts of protein. Hence, the nitrogenous wastes from protein breakdown were not converted to urea (as they should be generally in the liver) but into toxic substances that affected the brain. This was because inside the highly active liver cells (hepatocytes), something quite intricate and essential happens: the urea cycle. As I mentioned in the prologue, the urea cycle is a chain of chemical reactions within the liver cells that converts toxic ammonia waste generated from amino acids (the building blocks of protein) into urea, which is then excreted by the kidneys. The higher the protein content, the higher the generation of ammonia. If blood from the liver is diverted, then the chances of ammonia getting detoxified within the liver are unlikely, and the surge of excess ammonia into the system and finally into the brain through systemic blood circulation results in brain failure. For hepatic encephalopathy to occur, variables that enhanced ammonia production and redirected liver blood flow into the system are necessary. However, none of the dogs in these experiments had chronic liver disease or cirrhosis.

In 1932, two French clinician-scientists, Van Caulaert and Deviller, administered ammonia salts to persons with chronic liver disease. To their astonishment, the patients developed alterations in behaviour and insensibility. Some progressed to coma, demonstrating that ammonia loading in a system with a blighted liver resulted in brain dysfunction. How was this relevant to Ramesh's current clinical condition and underlying chronic liver disease?

~

Ramesh was getting worse back in the emergency room. As I spoke to Ravi about stabilizing his father on the ventilator, the physicians were inserting a breathing tube into Ramesh's trachea (windpipe) to safeguard his airways and prevent lung failure due to a rapidly progressing coma. After Ramesh was optimized, I contacted Ravi to briefly update him before transferring his father to the ICU, where the rest of this arduous struggle for survival would continue. The anxious son asked me only one question as he fought back tears: 'Doctor, please, could you tell me if my father will come off the ventilator?'

This is a common question doctors always hear—inside and outside the ICU, in the emergency room and inside the outpatient department. The question is apt, concerning and clichéd, but there is no honest answer. There never would be because 'medicine' is, and always will be, 'a science of uncertainty and an art of probability'.

I did not have answers but only feared that the responsibility would overburden me and, through me, the patient's family, and ultimately, it would crush us all under an excruciatingly emotive force that would hurt for a long time. The doctors at the ICU notified me that Ramesh's blood work was ready. A teetotaller with long-standing diabetes, well-controlled on regular medications, without any known drug or substance use, was suddenly fighting for his life on the ventilator. Infection screenings came back negative, and alcohol and toxicology screens also came back clean. His liver function tests were normal, except for a slight reduction in albumin, alongside a low platelet count (thrombocytopenia). The former meant that Ramesh's liver's ability to synthesize normal proteins was affected, and the latter revealed that his liver pressures were high.

To add to his woes, the liver's detoxification function was also affected since the blood ammonia levels were high. But Ramesh's liver was not failing, as he did not have jaundice. We all stepped back and looked at Ramesh's current clinical scenario. He had cirrhosis and sudden-onset but rapidly progressive high-ammonia-related brain failure without other known causes for the conditions. This was strange because, in cirrhosis, high ammonia and brain failure occur in the later stages of the disease, after liver failure has set in—that is, after the development of disease-related bleeding, fluid in the abdomen (ascites) and jaundice. But Ramesh had none of these, and he had presented with brain failure at first diagnosis. When a cirrhosis patient develops brain failure spontaneously—in the absence of advanced disease and the presence of a historically well-known precipitating factor, such as protein loading due to a meaty dinner—it is time to look for another culprit.

A Sanctuary Inside the Home

I reached home late that night. As my children surrounded me to show their new drawings and projects from school, I imagined one of my parents on that bed, like Ramesh, and my chest felt heavy. His face was etched into my brain.

I could not seem to forget his son's face either.

How would I cope?

What would I do?

What could I do?

As a family member of a sick patient, I would have nothing to offer but hope and prayer, I thought to myself. But I was the doctor here, and I had to do whatever it took to get that sick man off the ventilator and reunited with his small, profoundly loving family. I cleared my mind, and a warm bath later I was back inside the little bubble of sanctuary that my family provided—a little time off from the saddening reality into a small world of happiness that was mine. But like the inside of every other physician's mind, I subconsciously continued to think about getting Ramesh off the ventilator. My thoughts went deep into the history of medicine, as I intuitively flipped the pages from history on hepatic encephalopathy.

In 1954, the British physician, medical educator and pioneering liver disease specialist Dame Sheila Patricia Violet Sherlock and her colleagues observed a characteristic clinical situation among cirrhosis patients under their care. Some patients developed spontaneous episodes of abnormal behaviour, confusion and sleepiness that at times acutely progressed to coma, but responded to dietary protein withdrawal. The researchers performed detailed imaging of the abdomen of these patients. They found extensive, tortuous, snake-like newly formed blood vessels around the liver and other hollow organs that shunted blood away from the liver. They called the condition 'portal-systemic encephalopathy'. They defined it as a neuropsychiatric disorder that affected liver disease patients when a combination of nitrogenous wastes, such as ammonia, accumulated in the intestines in the presence of large shunts that bypassed blood away from the liver, resulting in ineffective detoxification. This portosystemic way of shunting away blood ensured that the blood bypassed the liver, missed detoxification and bathed the other organs, including the brain, in toxins.

As we've discussed earlier, ammonia has unfavourable effects on the brain cells (neurons). Significant ammonia levels can cause hepatic encephalopathy or brain dysfunction when it enters the brain cells. A complicated molecular reaction triggers micro-short circuits inside the neurons that cause electrical activity to slow down and the cells themselves to swell. However, it was not until almost three decades later that doctors at the University of Southern California, Los Angeles County Medical Center, headed by Dr K.C. Lam, correlated, without doubt, the presence of large portosystemic shunts and spontaneous brain dysfunction in liver disease patients.

~

The next day, back at the hospital, a CT scan imaging of Ramesh's abdomen was requested as soon as it became clear that he exhibited the classic characteristics that Dr Hahn documented in his dog experiments decades earlier, and similar to what Professor Sherlock described in her observed patients. A team of highly skilled nurses, a doctor experienced in the ICU and an anaesthesia consultant moved a critically unwell Ramesh (who was being ventilated by a machine) to the scan room, where the procedure was to be carried out. Ramesh's family, including Ravi, watched from across the imaging console through a glass pane as he moved back and forth inside the gigantic, hollow contraption that resembled a sophisticated, incomplete cave. It would hopefully provide answers to what was killing their loved one without warning. Ramesh had now been unconscious for more than seventy-two hours.

And then we found our answer.

The scan revealed a massive blood vessel, a portosystemic shunt, the size of a thickly meandering boa constrictor, siphoning blood away from Ramesh's liver into the central circulatory system. His brain was persistently washed by the ammonia and toxin-rich blood, powerfully enough to shut it down. A high-protein meal on that night had increased ammonia production, which the liver could not handle, and in the presence of a large shunt, the toxic nitrogenous wastes had slowly and steadily engulfed the patient's brain, short-circuiting neuronal functions and gradually causing Ramesh to lose cognition as he progressed through the stages of hepatic encephalopathy—exactly how it was described by Professor Morgagni 200 years ago.

The first step in treating brain dysfunction caused by high ammonia in patients with cirrhosis was to lower the ammonia levels. Several medications were developed to address this, the most important of which was lactulose, a delightfully sweet but non-absorbable flavoured sugary syrup first produced in 1929. As bacteria completely metabolize lactulose in the large intestine, there are no major systemic side effects. The history of lactulose is fascinating. It was first used to treat brain failure in chronic liver disease patients in 1966. At the time, researchers believed that the preferential increase in a specific bacterium in the large intestine called *Lactobacillus,* which lacked an enzyme called urease, was the reason for its benefits. Urease aids in breaking urea into ammonia, which then enters the systemic circulation. However, as *Lactobacillus* levels rise, urea splitting and ammonia production decline, improving brain function. Moreover, in animal and human studies, scientists discovered that even if *Lactobacillus* levels did not rise, ammonia generation dropped significantly and brain dysfunction improved.

To explain the effectiveness of lactulose, a professor of medicine at the University of Göttingen, Germany, started to look inside the large intestine for answers. Johannes Bircher knew that bacteria in the large bowel broke down lactulose into lactic acid and acetic acid. Because these acids lower the pH inside the large colon, the contents of the large bowel became acidified. Ammonia (toxic and free) was converted to ammonium (non-toxic salt) in an acidic environment, which could not be absorbed back into the circulation and was thus excreted in faeces—lowering ammonia levels in the bowels and blood. But that was not the end of lactulose's magic. There was also another mechanism that Professor Bircher found. When the large intestine became acidic (that is, the acidity was less than 6.2) ammonia in the blood flowed into the lumen. Bircher referred to this as 'acid dialysis of the colon' because lactulose reduced significant intestinal absorption and increased intestinal ammonia excretion, thereby improving brain function.

The Dying Patient and a Living One

As Ramesh was on a ventilator, sedated and relaxed to protect his airways, a tube was inserted through his nose into his stomach, and 150 ml of lactulose was given daily in three divided doses, along with lactulose enemas twice daily—an aggressive attempt to wash out all the ammonia from the system and to enforce a redeeming 'acid dialysis of the colon', as Bircher described it. And it was fruitful. Within a day, Ramesh began to move his limbs and was awake enough to bite at the tube connected to the ventilator, which supplied oxygen to his lungs.

We persisted. We rained down every therapeutic attempt at lowering ammonia levels for more than five days, but Ramesh showed no signs of further improvement. This was concerning because the longer the patient was on mechanical ventilation, the greater the risk of infection and other grave complications. He was on the ventilator because we were out of options. We needed to get him off the machine as soon as possible. The large portosystemic shunt that was bypassing all of Ramesh's blood away from his shrunken liver was challenging to beat medically. However, medical science is not one to accept defeat so soon. Since scientific medicine is dynamic, when one door closes, another one opens. It always finds a way. It is uplifting, fulfilling and ultimately satisfying. So we looked for ways to beat the shunt when medications failed.

Dr Sherif Hanna of the Sunnybrook Medical Center in Toronto, Canada, and his colleagues speculated in 1981—the same year that Dr Lam demonstrated that large shunts could cause severe and recurrent brain failure in cirrhosis patients—that closing the large blood vessel in patients with recurrent or uncontrolled shunt-related brain failure could improve detoxification and awaken patients. In August, the group published findings on (surgical) shunt closure in seven patients with severe or recurrent ammonia-induced brain dysfunction, reporting complete recovery and reduced ammonia levels in four patients as predicted.

It took over three decades to publish studies of the closure of shunts in patients with portosystemic collaterals using non-surgical techniques. A multicentre European study found that occluding large shunts in cirrhosis patients, with medically difficult-to-control brain failure, using radiological techniques—similar to angioplasty for heart blocks—resulted in significantly improved outcomes. With this evidence, we decided to proceed with Ramesh, who was now in and out of a cyclical coma.

It was not easy to block the monstrous shunt. A surgical block was impossible because Ramesh would not survive an open surgery. This was where the importance of another subset of doctors came into play: interventional radiologists or, in hospital vernacular, the 'IR'.

The 'IR gang' could access any organ system through the peripheral blood vessels—arteries or veins—with no cuts or openings and no scars. Once the task was completed, there would be no evidence that they had ever been there. It was like a 'surgical strike' (but without the surgery) against specific medically difficult-to-treat disease conditions, such as cirrhosis-related shunt syndrome.

The IR was notified about the patient, and after a quick review of the clinical situation, anaesthesia requirements and levels of organ support, Ramesh was duly transported from the ICU to the IR department on the eighth day of his admission. The IR doctors inserted a wire through his neck vein, guiding it through the larger veins in the chest and abdomen to access the large shunt, which they then completely blocked using platinum-based coils that induced clotting.

After the procedure, Ramesh was transferred back to the ICU. The doctors there closely monitored Ramesh for signs of improvement or clinical deterioration. To their great surprise, they discovered that his ammonia levels were drastically reducing. Ramesh woke up on the fourth day following the procedure. He woke up confused, but his eyes opened spontaneously to commands. He struggled, dazed by what was happening around him and was trying to get the large tube out of his windpipe.

'Relax, Ramesh,' said the senior ICU physician. 'You are fine, and we will remove this tube from you as soon as possible. But you must help us understand that you can breathe on your own.'

Ramesh nodded in agreement.

We had brought Ramesh's son and wife with us. They stood by his bedside, staring at him. Ramesh's eyes welled up with tears as Ravi squeezed his father's hand. If the gazes could talk, they would tell the story of doubt, pain, death and hope, made possible by scientific observations, practice and experiments—on dogs and humans—that woke up a dying man. Ramesh was eventually weaned off the ventilator, moved out of the ICU and discharged home after a remarkable three-week hospital stay.

On the day of discharge, as I was saying goodbye to a new patient in the outpatient department, Ramesh and his son walked in.

I stood up and shook their hands.

Ramesh gripped my left elbow and stared at me, saying nothing.

But I understood the passing thoughts that lit up inside his brain and smiled at him, to which he responded, 'Thank you, sir.'

~

The phone rang as I saw them go out the door and I returned to my seat.

It was from the emergency room. I heard words from the other end and became concerned, as the on-call doctor spoke frantically. I had the impression that a dark cloud was hovering above me. Something sinister was on its way.

'What is it?' I inquired.

'Could you please get to the emergency room as soon as possible?' he asked hastily.

'Is the patient deeply ill?'

'Yes, and it is a little girl. Not jaundiced but appears unstable. Please come quickly,' the emergency physician hurried me, his words stumbling.

He then added, 'But there is a man too, and he is in a coma and on the ventilator. You must see him first. We will handle the admission of the child.'

Before he could finish the sentence, I hung up and rushed out of the door, taking the steps down to the emergency department, unsure of the battle ahead.

Riddle Me This

The Invisible Enemy

I walked up to the middle-aged woman, who looked palpably worried. This was the third time her husband had been admitted to the ICU, and each time had been worse than the previous admission. This time, he was in a coma, and the reasons for his recurrent altered behaviour remained elusive. There was only one clue: he had cirrhosis. Shankar, the woman's husband, had been diagnosed with cirrhosis only a couple of months back. At the time, he had swelling in both feet, and an evaluation revealed the presence of low platelets in his blood work and the features of cirrhosis on imaging scans. Back then, he had absolutely no complications associated with cirrhosis.

Complications of cirrhosis come in stages. Stages 1 and 2 feature changes associated with cirrhosis and high liver pressure (portal hypertension), while Stages 3 and 4 are when clinical events in the form of various complications start as part of the natural history of the disease. These include ascites and blood vomiting or the passage of tarry black stools. In the stages beyond these, patients develop features of liver failure—such as jaundice (defined as total bilirubin levels >3 mg/dL) and brain failure (hepatic encephalopathy). In the natural history of cirrhosis, brain failure is expected to happen only in the advanced stages and is dangerous because its occurrence independently predicts early death. Patients with hepatic encephalopathy progress through various stages, starting from slight memory loss and difficulty in simple calculation tasks to slurred speech, confusion and, finally, coma. Almost 30–45 per cent of cirrhosis patients experience brain failure during their illness. Diagnosing hepatic encephalopathy is easy—it means ruling out the presence of other causes of brain failure or neurological dysfunction such as stroke, brain infections, brain tumours, intoxication and trauma to the brain. So essentially, brain failure due to cirrhosis is a diagnosis of exclusion. Once this is diagnosed, the most crucial part is looking for the trigger of the brain failure.

In the emergency room, Shankar was being put on the ventilator because he was in a coma, the last stage of hepatic encephalopathy, and the chances of aspiration of saliva into his lungs were very high, and lung failure was imminent. They were a small, loving, close-knit family: a father, a mother and a daughter. Their daughter was twenty-two years old and engaged to a gentleman, and their wedding was to happen in three months. It was after her engagement that Shankar had been diagnosed with cirrhosis, and within two months of his diagnosis, he was admitted thrice with brain failure. Now, he was in a coma, and she was worried that on her wedding day, she would miss her beloved Appa, as she called her father.

My colleagues took a detailed history. Shankar was a teetotaller, a gentleman who followed doctor's orders to the T and worked hard to make ends meet for the well-being of his family. He was heavily invested in making his family lead a comfortable life. He was overweight but avoided recreational or prescription drug use. The first time he got sick, it started with him mistaking the living room for the bathroom and, in a confused state, he had been getting ready to urinate on the living room floor. Disoriented and in altered behaviour, he was rushed to a nearby hospital, where he was diagnosed with brain failure associated with his cirrhosis and treated accordingly. The second encephalopathy episode attacked him again without warning and came three weeks later—this time, he was disoriented while riding his bike and crashed into a street pole very close to his home. There were no brain injuries and, again, treatment for brain failure associated with cirrhosis was initiated, which improved his condition drastically, and he was discharged home uneventfully.

The third episode, the current one, had landed him in a coma and on the ventilator in our ICU. Time was running out, and we had to find out the reason behind his current and recurrent brain failure. To make things worse, his liver functions were perfectly within the expected range, and his cirrhosis condition was only on Stage 2—brain failure was not an expected complication in this stable stage.

What is causing it? we all pondered.

When a patient with stable cirrhosis presents with recurrent brain failure in the absence of identifiable causes for precipitation of the encephalopathy, we call it 'spontaneous hepatic encephalopathy'. As we waited for the blood reports, we sent Shankar for a CT scan of the brain and abdomen, to help us identify an essential cause for his recurrent spontaneous brain failure episodes—a condition associated with cirrhosis, called the portosystemic shunt syndrome.

As you may remember from earlier discussions, portosystemic shunts are hugely dilated and enlarged veins that form inside the abdomen in patients with cirrhosis when the liver pressure increases, as the liver shrinks and blood flow into the liver gets hampered. These portosystemic shunts ferry the blood away from the liver and go straight into the system, dumping all toxic wastes on the brain. We saw this in Ramesh in our previous story, but he had a favourable outcome.

Even though we expected Shankar to have such large shunts, surprisingly, we did not find any on the CT scans, and portosystemic shunts as the cause for recurrent brain failure was essentially ruled out. Meanwhile, his blood reports were uploaded to the computer system, and more surprisingly, everything was normal.

Except for two small things.

Shankar's potassium levels were very low, and his blood ammonia was raised. Low potassium levels, hypokalemia in medical terms, were a significant risk factor that precipitated brain failure in cirrhosis patients. Finally, we had a reason for Shankar's current brain failure episode. The treatment was simple. Correct the potassium levels in the blood, and Shankar would be all right. When potassium levels drop, the capacity for urea synthesis reduces in the liver (urea generation occurs in the liver through the urea cycle reaction within the liver cells), leading to increased blood ammonia, which, as we know, causes brain failure in cirrhosis. But also, when potassium goes low, it triggers the conversion of the amino acid glutamine in the kidneys into excess ammonia in the blood. The excess ammonia enters circulation, reaches the brain and causes encephalopathy. To control this, we started potassium correction for Shankar and told his wife and daughter that things would be all right, and that they had no reason to worry for now. However, we did not yet have genuine reasons for Shankar's recurrent brain failure. We asked the family about the reasons that other doctors who treated Shankar for the first and second attacks of encephalopathy had given them.

'It was high ammonia,' said his wife.

'But potassium was also low, Amma,' the daughter chipped in.

I sat up, listened and asked them again.

'Was potassium low both times?'

They nodded in unison.

'Can I see the previous discharge summaries?'

That is when we saw something very intriguing. Shankar, during all his three attacks of brain failure, had low potassium levels in his blood. But the million-dollar question was: Why was his potassium going low repeatedly?

We knew it was time. Time we stopped being super-specialists and got back to the heart and soul of real clinical medicine: internal medicine. Back to the mothership. Back to being generalists.

Hiding in Plain Sight

The causes for low potassium are vast. But we were only interested in the causes of recurrent low potassium in Shankar. To get to it, we needed the help of the best thing ever in clinical medicine practice: algorithms.

So we pulled up the approach to recurrent low potassium in a patient algorithm to figure out how and why Shankar was losing potassium.

Firstly, we looked at his drugs list. A host of drugs can lower potassium in the human body, but Shankar was not on any such medications. So we moved to the rest of the algorithm to determine why this happened. Investigations required us to look at two things in Shankar. One, if the potassium was lost through kidneys or due to non-kidney causes; and two, the percentage (fractional) of potassium excretion in the urine. Following these two investigations, we discovered that Shankar's urine potassium was relatively high and his blood was alkaline (called metabolic alkalosis). At admission to our hospital, his blood pressure was higher, which was also true for every other admission in the previous hospitals. The major potassium-handling hormone, aldosterone, secreted by adrenal glands was low.

This was strange.

Low potassium.

High blood pressure.

Alkaline blood.

All were common at every admission.

High aldosterone levels can cause these, but remember that in Shankar's case, the levels of aldosterone were low. This condition is called pseudo (or false) hyperaldosteronism. This disorder mimics high aldosterone levels when, in fact, aldosterone levels are either low or normal, and can happen due to rare causes, which include various types of diseases that affect the glands that make and release hormones; certain factors in the diet; and, rarely, genetic causes. Shankar's clinical presentation did not fit right with any genetic diseases or hormone-related disorders. We were now left with only three other causes that could cause 'pseudo hyperaldosteronism'.

One, licorice consumption.

Two, the use of a drug called carbenoxolone.

Or three, high consumption of grapefruits.

We got back to the family, who were still waiting patiently for the mechanically ventilated Shankar to get better. Very clearly and slowly, I asked his wife and daughter about his dietary and drug habits. They denied excessive consumption of licorice or drugs, and even grapefruit intake.

We were back to square one and were indeed lost. Without finding the exact cause of recurrent low potassium levels, Shankar was still at risk for brain failure even if he did survive the current critical episode. He was a cirrhosis patient, and the chances of him getting through to attend his daughter's wedding seemed bleak. This depressed us, and we did not know how to get through it.

One day, while I was seeing my routine patients in the outpatient department, my office staff notified me that Shankar's wife wanted to meet with me. I allowed her the time because I knew we had done everything possible to get to the root cause of her husband's condition. The wife walked in and looked at me, and I composed myself to apologize to her because we thought we could do it, but we had failed her.

'Dear doctor, I have been thinking for a long time about your diet queries,' she told me. 'And even though he did not consume any of those fruits you had mentioned, he was taking some laxative powder.'

I sat up, curious, and asked her the name of the powder. She said she did not know because he had kept it inside the bathroom shelf, and she never looked at it.

Cirrhosis patients are usually prescribed lactulose, a safe laxative that helps them pass soft stools and reduce blood ammonia. Lactulose did not suit Shankar because a common side effect was excessive bloating. Hence, he had chosen another laxative option on his own, the name of which only he knew.

'Only Shankar knows about it and can tell us what he was taking back home, and for that, he has to be weaned off the ventilator,' I told the wife.

Then we focused every bit of our energy on getting Shankar off of the ventilator. The only person who could tell us the diagnosis was the patient himself.

We went all out treating his brain failure as per evidence and by the book. Even though it took us more than a week to get to our goal, we finally weaned Shankar off the ventilator. His voice was raspy, and he was weak. His swallowing was affected, and he was dazed. The ICU nursing team did an intense and immense job of rehabilitating Shankar so that we could shift him out of the unit. After another week in the ICU, Shankar was finally moved to a hospital room. His potassium levels had normalized, and his blood pressure improved. His blood was no longer alkaline. That day finally came when, on rounds, I could ask him about the powder he was consuming as a laxative.

Kayam Churna is a traditional Ayurvedic medicine used to treat constipation. It contains senna leaves, known herbal laxatives, and, more importantly, Yashtimadhu (in Sanskrit) or *Glycyrrhiza glabra*—also called licorice.

Licorice consumption has been very strongly associated with low potassium. Excessive licorice intake is a well-known cause of high blood pressure or hypertension. A compound in licorice called glycyrrhizin inhibits an enzyme in the kidney, causing a rise in the levels of the hormone cortisol, which leads to loss of potassium and increased blood pressure. The main issue with using a natural herbal product containing senna laxatives is that they reach a limiting threshold for effective action in the body. Then they do not work unless doses are increased.

Across two months of daily use, Shankar had slowly and steadily increased his Kayam use, which led to severe potassium loss, leading to hypokalemia, which then precipitated his recurrent hepatic encephalopathy or brain failure. Licorice herbal products must be taken with caution or not be taken at all, especially in high-risk patient groups, such as those with cirrhosis. They may appear and are marketed as safe, but the truth is bitter. They have never been completely safe.

After spending almost three weeks in the hospital, Shankar was discharged. Back home, the first thing he did was throw the rest of the Kayam Churna out of the window.

A few months later, a teary-eyed Shankar watched his daughter dance with her husband on her wedding day.

He sent me a message on that day.

It did not contain any words.

But only two emoticons: <3 and :-).

It has been more than three years, and Shankar has never had another episode of brain failure since the last time we fought for him, and he fought on the ventilator.

I showed my team the message, and we all looked at it without saying any words to each other. Then we returned to our hospital duties to take care of the new patients who had come to us.

The words of Jonathan Harnisch echoed in my mind: 'The strongest people are not those who show strength in front of the world but those who fight and win battles that others do not know anything about.'

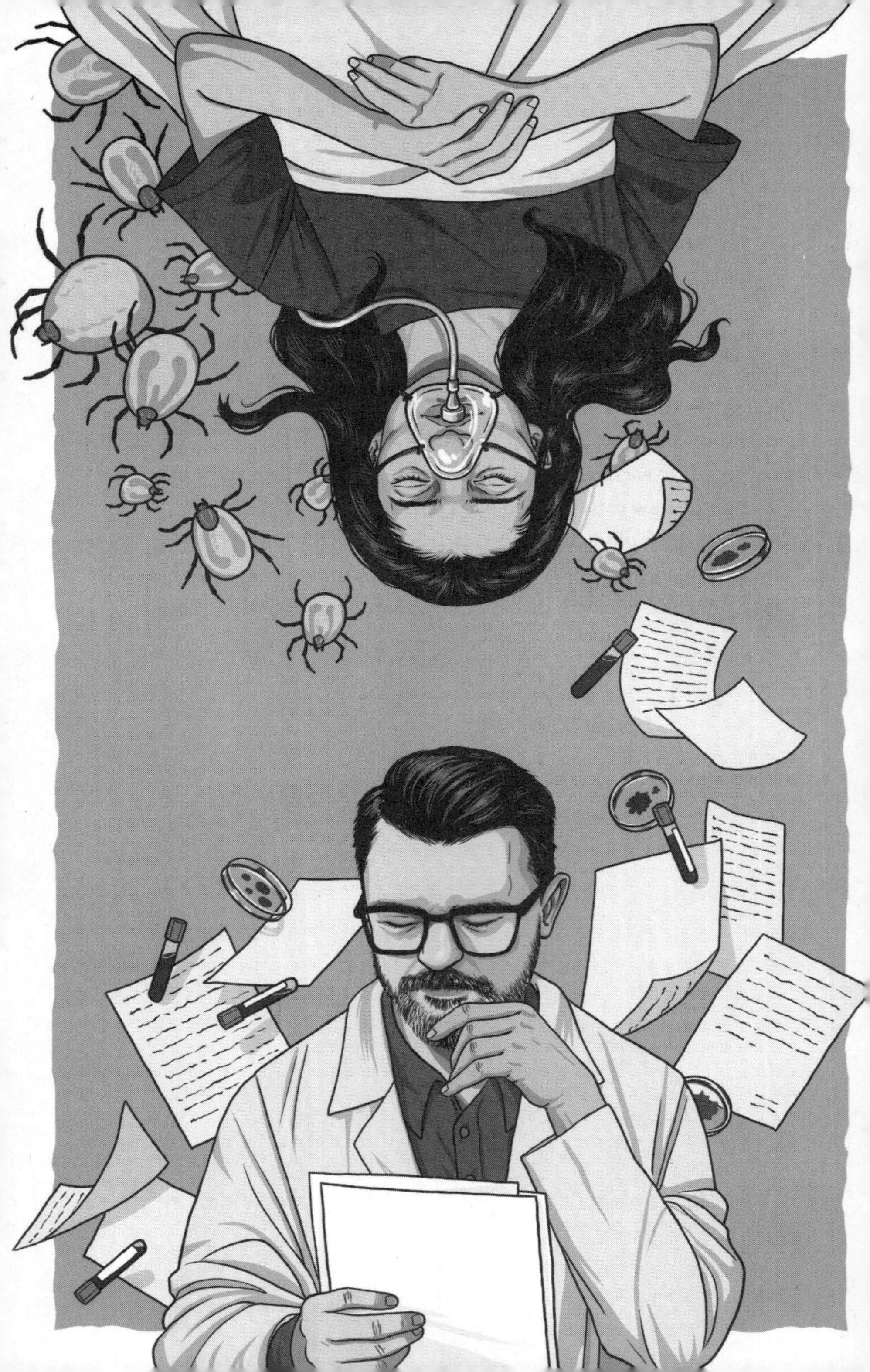

CHAPTER 5

This Yellow-Tailed Oriole

Into the World of Infectious Liver Diseases

The Critter

'It is during our darkest moments that we must focus to see the light.'
—Aristotle

The Mother of a Child

One moment I am back at that little rice field that surrounded my home in the quaint little village in that quiet little suburb. I am in my fourth-grade year, back from school, and I feel free. I am leaning on that brick fence with the perfect height. The breeze blows gently through my hair, on my face, and I feel the cold as it touches the drops of sweat on my forehead. There are no walls. The water below glistens and I see little fish with silver spots on their heads move under the surface. My brother and sisters are running around. My mother calls out to me for a small glass of warm chocolate malt drink.

The next moment, I am inside a room. There are walls around and the sound of wailing. People in scrubs and whites run helter-skelter. The place has no breeze, but it's cooler because it is air-conditioned. My hair does not move, and I am not really sweating. But then, I am sweating too. I am not free. My mind is bound. It has been trained to focus. I see the rice field at a great distance, but I am unable to focus there. I let go of the breeze and embrace the walls.

I looked at the young mother lying on the hospital bed. She was shivering and her fever was spiking. When the fever settled, she would sweat buckets on the bedsheet like someone had opened a faucet. But there was something more sinister afoot. Her liver functions were deranged. And they were climbing. Her baby girl was waiting back home, and her father was troubled. I was faced with an unknown foe, so tiny, yet so powerful it nearly broke me.

Nearly.

~

The young patient, Silvia, was a happy new mother to a one-year-old daughter. Her husband was back in the Middle East after spending six months at home, working hard to provide for the close family of three. Everything was set in stone, and things looked great. But a week ago, Silvia had started to lose her appetite. What followed were waves of high-spiking fever. Some bouts were so disabling and fatiguing that Silvia looked at her one-year-old as a burden, and she felt unimaginably bad about such disruptive, vile thoughts. All she wanted to do was sleep. When she did eventually sleep, she would wake up the next day as if she had not slept at all, because the lethargy was crippling. However, the lethargy was not the worst. Terrible, deep-seated body aches and drenching sweats were ruining her mental health. She would eat very little. Her father called and, seeing what state she was in, paid for a temporary full-time house help to keep the routines rolling. Silvia looked like Death to her father as she lay in bed most of the time, day in and day out.

What they thought was a passing viral flu did not pass, even after three days of medication use for symptom control. On the fourth day, Silvia was rushed to a nearby clinic, where the doctors ran initial tests.

Her white blood cell count, a marker of severe infection, was normal, and her liver test results were only mildly elevated—'Nothing much to worry about,' assured the emergency physician on duty. They gave her injectable paracetamol, and her fever and body aches settled to tolerable levels. After a day of observation, Silvia was sent home with a short course of round-the-clock paracetamol, and the doctor advised her to keep herself well hydrated. 'It was most likely a passing viral flu,' came the reassurance again at discharge.

But that night was terrible. The sweeping fevers were back, and the drenching sweats followed. All the pain and fever medications were being overwhelmed by the symptoms. When Silvia looked like Death again, her father rushed her to another hospital the same night. This time, a bigger one, with specialists who would help them get to the bottom of the mysterious fever.

Silvia was admitted. And her blood work was done again. New tests revealed that her white blood cell counts were slightly elevated, and her liver tests were still rising. The liver enzymes (aspartate transaminase and alanine transaminase) were now in the 200s—they were in the 60s a day before (normal is usually below 40). However, Silvia was on fever medication round-the-clock, and the new doctors in charge thought this could be the reason for an increase in liver enzymes. As they waited for other results to return, a new symptom started to haunt their patient: vomiting. She could not stand the sight of food and would retch immediately. There were no contents to her vomitus because she hardly ate anything. The intravenous fluids kept her hydrated.

Headaches followed. She said it felt as if someone was thumping her head with a jackhammer, and her eyes turned red. Daily surveillance blood tests were going haywire, especially the liver function tests. The liver enzymes were sky-high, but the jaundice parameters were not so. The doctors were sure now. High-grade fever, no jaundice, but abnormal liver enzymes, severe body aches, headaches and vomiting—the diagnosis was so clear and straightforward. The weather was perfect for this. It was the rainy season.

Ancient Foes

In medical encyclopaedias written during the Chinese Jin (or Chin) Dynasty period (265–420 CE), physician monks refer to a disease called 'water poison'. This was peculiarly associated with increased flying insects in the vicinity, especially after rains. Even though this was the first record of this disease, humankind's understanding of what caused it and how it spread came hundreds of centuries later. In the African lands, the Swahili people called it 'ki denga pepo', describing a sudden, cramp-like seizure that they thought was due to an evil spirit. But those affected with it were experiencing common symptoms: high fever, headache, severe bone and body aches and significant fatigue. But it was not until the 1780s that people started noticing large outbreaks of this disease, with similar characteristics having been described ages earlier.

During the 1780 and 1789 epidemics of fevers, a physician from Philadelphia, Benjamin Rush, described a fever that was crippling all patients it affected with painful fatigue. He called it 'break-bone fever'. Into the 1820s, physicians realized that it was like what was described in ancient Chinese literature. From the African continent, 'ki denga pepo' was replaced by its short form, dengue. Only in 1943 did Ren Kimura and Susumu Hotta first identify and isolate the causative agent of dengue, a virus, by injecting the serum of soldiers suffering from break-bone fever into the feet of suckling mice.

As clinicians and researchers kept studying dengue and its impact on humans, they identified another vital aspect of this ancient disease: dengue hepatitis. A severe form of liver inflammation sometimes affected those suffering from dengue, which was peculiar. It was associated with a lower presence of jaundice but sky-high liver-enzyme elevation on blood tests. The onset of jaundice in dengue fever was a bad sign. Sometimes, the liver injury was so damning that people died due to acute liver failure with the onset of brain failure, along with the development of jaundice and thinning of the blood due to the condition.

With this in mind, the doctors started hydrating Silvia with large boluses of intravenous fluids, a mainstay in the treatment of dengue, while they waited for the reports to come.

But there was an issue.

Results for dengue were negative, and the doctors were stumped.

Then, something new.

Silvia's eyes were now turning a milder tinge of yellow. The liver tests revealed that jaundice was setting in, and her liver enzymes were now almost ten times the upper limit of normal. She was lethargic, fatigued and still hardly ate. Silvia asked for her baby daughter from time to time, and her father, the designated bystander, affirmed that she was well at home. Silvia mumbled in her sleep every night about her daughter, and the older man could not bear it. What if everything went wrong? What if the worst happened? Even in the face of hope, the aged father prepared for the worst—a human conditioning so complex that his mind was thrown into chaos. Silvia was shifted to the ICU, where other doctors would do what they were supposed to do under exceptional circumstances—keep patients alive until the primary team could figure out what was killing them.

Since the liver tests were worsening daily, paracetamol use was rationed to control only the worst fevers, while cold sponging was initiated to bring the temperature down. Larger doses and longer duration of paracetamol use can harm the liver. Was the jaundice due to paracetamol toxicity? The ICU doctors ruled it out by checking levels of the medication in Silvia's blood and finding that they were within range. Silvia's husband, who worked in the Middle East, was now distraught. He had just spent some quality time with the mother and their newborn and got back to work. His privilege to fly down again and be with Silvia was not part of his reality, since he had taken an extended leave of absence and had just joined a new company. He kept calling his father-in-law multiple times a day to check on Silvia, only to be disappointed with the news that she was holding on, but there was no hope, and that now she was in the ICU. Silvia's father was burdened.

What would he tell the family if she got sicker and everything went dark?

How would they manage the little child?

How could they cope?

He started to go down the rabbit hole of depression and uncertainty, as everything seemed unreal. The mountains of investigations done at the hospital seemed like a conspiracy to him. Maybe the doctors knew what affected Silvia but did not want the treatment to end early. They were milking the situation and gaining from the family's ordeal—or so the family thought. At some point, for Silvia's father, everything seemed like an opportunist's dream come true and everyone was a villain. When doctors came in to discuss the same situation repeatedly, he would give them the cold shoulder and remain aloof. His demeanour would change, and the doctors would feel it too. The whole environment was turning toxic, and so was Silvia's condition.

~

Disease is the ultimate equalizer. It doesn't care about your happiness, wealth, resources to fight it or future plans; it strikes without warning, forcing everyone to play by its rules. In an instant, life can shift from normal to critical, which is why the present matters more than anything. Live fully today—whether it's a task, a trip, a conversation, a forgotten greeting or a long-overdue goodbye. Because today is all we truly have. This was precisely what the intensivists' treatment of Silvia was doing. They started working on her more aggressively. They went at it, step by step, piece by piece. Looking at every single infection, from detail to detail.

Where did they get it wrong? Did they miss something? Silvia had sudden onset hepatitis, which was now progressing to jaundice. Dengue was out, and they knew it.

What about the other possibilities? They started with the most common ones.

As we discussed earlier, jaundice first attracted attention over 5,000 years ago. Hippocrates called it icterus, after a bird with golden plumage. Ancient tradition held that placing this bird near a patient would draw out the yellowness, healing the human while the bird died.

For centuries, the cause for jaundice remained a mystery. Ancient Sumerians blamed a liver-attacking devil named Ahhazu. Later, Hippocrates described the clinical course of epidemic jaundice, though the only treatment was honey and water. By 752 CE, Pope Zachary noted that isolation curbed the spread, as the 'impure' patients were separated. During the American Civil War (1861–65) and the World Wars, the disease became known as 'Campaign Jaundice', a morbid affliction looming over soldiers in their barracks.

The path to understanding the cause can be found in botany. In 1898, following work on tobacco plant diseases, Martinus Beijerinck coined the term 'virus'. By 1932, the first human virus—yellow fever—was isolated. But the liver remained an enigma until 1946, when microbiologist Frederick Ogden MacCallum distinguished between 'infectious hepatitis' (Type A) and 'serum hepatitis' (Type B).

Sometimes, in the quest for truth, humans go to dark places. When curiosity overwhelms morality and achievements surpass integrity, bad medicine is born. This was grimly illustrated at the Willowbrook State School in Staten Island, New York, starting in 1956. For fourteen years, children with mental health disabilities—many of them autistic—became unwilling subjects in a devilish experiment to track the development of the viral infection. In a horrifying breach of trust, these children were intentionally infected, either by direct injection of infectious material or by being made to drink chocolate milk mixed with faeces from infected peers. While these studies provided data distinguishing the two types of transmission—the shorter incubation of the faeces-to-oral route versus the longer blood-borne route—it remains a dark chapter in which the pursuit of science eclipsed the sanctity of human welfare.

Discoveries accelerated in 1963 when geneticist Baruch Blumberg identified the 'Australia antigen'. After a lab accident involving his colleague, the link between this antigen and serum hepatitis was confirmed, leading to the identification of the hepatitis B virus in 1970. Shortly after, in 1977, Stephen Feinstone identified the culprit behind infectious hepatitis in stool specimens: hepatitis A.

Medical science, however, has a bittersweet habit; it does not rest. In the 1970s, researchers hunted for a 'non-A, non-B' agent that caused chronic liver damage after transfusions. Using advanced molecular techniques, a team led by Michael Houghton and Harvey Alter finally identified hepatitis C, a virus that rarely caused acute jaundice but silently damaged the liver.

Meanwhile, a water-borne mystery was unfolding in India and China. Massive outbreaks resembled hepatitis A but tested negative. In 1983, Russian virologist Mikhail Balayan consumed infected faecal material, reproducing the disease in himself to prove the existence of a new agent. In 1990, using molecular identification, this virus was finally named hepatitis E.

Viral hepatitis is the most common diagnosis of acute onset hepatitis in a country like India. In north India, the hepatitis E virus predominates, while in the south, it is hepatitis A.

Review and repeat tests for acute onset viral hepatitis were, unfortunately, not contributory in Silvia. After another forty-eight hours of testing and treating for symptoms, Silvia was nowhere near better, and there was something dark brooding around the corner.

The ICU doctors realized it, and it sent shivers down their spines.

It was puzzling and terrifying. They were now looking at something that was considered most sinister in clinical medicine. A terrible condition that would drain resources—both financial and human—and leave everyone exhausted by the end of it all, sometimes without an answer, or at times with an answer that had no further solutions, ending with the patient dying. They called it a 'fever of unknown origin' or

FUO; it required the utmost focus. It required expertise to connect the dots. A relentless fever could be due to anything from a passing seasonal flu to a dreadful blood cancer that could kill.

But Silvia's fever was peculiar. All the while, one aspect stood out in our investigations. One player never left the field in this game of life and death inside that ICU. The headaches were less, and the fatigue had reduced. The bone aches were slightly better. But one organ system was consistently crying out loud: the liver.

This was FUO with acute hepatitis and jaundice. On what had started out as a routine day at the outpatient department, there was now a hostile situation developing in the ICU, and a baby girl was waiting for the patient back home. My team briefly reviewed the medical problem and sent me a message about the patient's condition. Silvia was not looking good, and there was a lot at stake. This was not a simple 'suggest-act-and-go' medical consult but something that required much more time and effort, and a significant investment of brainstorming sessions. It was a task that looked easy—fever with hepatitis—but one that could remain incomplete with the death of the patient.

Within three hours of the review, Silvia was transferred to the liver unit, empowering us to be her primary care physicians.

The New Vanguard

We looked at Silvia. She looked toxic, dehydrated and cripplingly lethargic. Dengue had been ruled out, and her platelet counts had not fallen as expected. It could not have been tuberculosis because the time frame was too short, the clinical presentation unconvincing and a very critical aspect of tuberculosis diagnosis—the imaging—wholly negative. We looked at the tests the previous team and the intensivists had performed. All causes for viral hepatitis were effectively ruled out. Other infections that could have secondarily affected the liver to cause jaundice, the parasitic illnesses malaria and leptospirosis (a severe bacterial disease that spreads through the urine of infected animals such as rodents, dogs and farm animals, which causes the individual to develop kidney failure and bleeding, along with high spiking fevers and severe loss of appetite and body aches) were both negative. A widespread typhoid infection caused by the bacterium *Salmonella typhi*, which spreads through contaminated food and water, was also negative, as Silvia had never had food out on the streets, away from her home environment. Again, we looked at prescription drugs, medications, HDS and other traditional and folk remedies that could have potentially affected the liver. Since Silvia was lactating and she had only very recently stopped breastfeeding her child, she was reluctant to consume drugs and supplements, and was not on any such medications anyway. This effectively ruled out drug-induced liver injury. She was a teetotaller too.

We then looked at the pattern of her fever. In clinical medicine, fever may come with specific patterns that help clinch the diagnosis. Common viral and bacterial infections usually have a continuous or intermittent fever. In contrast, certain types of fever may come only once a day (with certain types of malaria); or with two distinct daily peaks (as seen in rare diseases such as leishmaniasis, a vector-borne disease that is transmitted by sandflies and caused by a parasitic protozoan called Leishmania); or periodical fevers that come and go in a few days, weeks or even months (notable in lymphoma); or fevers with two different phases during the same spike (notable in various other common and rare infections). Another type of fever is undulant fever, in which the temperature rises gradually and falls, like a wave, over days to weeks, which is seen in a disease called brucellosis (caused by a bacterium that infects people when they are in contact with infected animals or animal products, such as unpasteurized dairy).

Silvia's fever patterns were not well-defined. During the early period, it was intermittent; later, continuous; and then the pattern was disrupted with paracetamol for many days. We were back to square one because a deep review of the fever patterns in Silvia did not yield the solutions we thought it would. So as not to be biased with only infections, we also looked at tests that gave the possibility of fever arising from non-infectious causes—including systemic inflammatory diseases, such as autoimmune disorders; rheumatic illness; rare causes that affected hormonal glands, such as a high-functioning thyroid gland; and other systemic immunological diseases, as well as cancer. The previous team had drained out much of the testing resources to no avail. We were stuck with a highly feverish patient with worsening liver tests, and every commonly identifiable cause—from infectious, non-infectious and cancerous points of view—were all effectively ruled out. Even tests for rare viruses that cause fever and affect the liver returned negative. These included the Epstein–Barr virus, Cytomegalovirus, Adenovirus, Norovirus and many others tested through a special multiplex virus assessment. Infection involving the heart valves, called infectious endocarditis, also came back negative.

We did not want to repeat the tests, and blanket testing for everything meant that more money would have to be spent. In the two hospitals where Silvia was admitted, including ours, repeated testing and imaging for the known and regionally common infections, as well as advanced molecular testing, had already drained much money from the family. Silvia's father was getting impatient daily. This meant that every next step we took had to be purposeful.

We took a step back and reassessed the crucial points. There were two aspects: one's history of travel and rare infections that could also affect the liver. Silvia denied any recent travel. She was always home. Rare infections that affect the liver, apart from all the ones we had already ruled out, were only a few. We wrote them down based on published literature. Most of these infections were either spread by animals, tiny rodents or insects, or were due to travel and subsequent poisoning from water, food and other environmental sources. They were region-specific, so we looked at each of them in detail from a clinical-history point of view, and only focused on those that involved the liver.

The tests were sent out. One last drill. Antibiotics were upgraded because the fever spikes kept coming and going in waves; and her heart rate sometimes went through the roof, and the rhythm and rate became worryingly irregular. She was getting sicker but was oriented to place and person, not time. Apart from growing anxious, her father was now becoming furious. Money was drained from one side for many specialized investigations, and the liver was repeatedly assaulted from the other.

As Silvia's case dragged on in uncertainty, the fear that she might never return to her little daughter consumed me—stealing my sleep and appetite and dulling the joy of weekends and family. Each negative report made it harder to face her father, and I feared tensions with the family might erupt into conflict. Twice a day, I repeated the same grim updates, my words feeling hollow. The weight of it all drained me—mentally, emotionally and physically. Even the simple comfort of coming home to my wife's warm banana fritters and pot of hot coffee lost its meaning; the snacks went cold, the coffee remained unfinished. My team and I were stretched thin, living on edge, as each new report brought more despair, and even facing the family became a burden I dreaded.

One day, I got a call from the hospital's central lab.

A blood test we had sent to an outside lab for a rare disease had returned positive. I hurried to the ICU where Silvia was recovering from another bout of fever and lay exhausted. The ICU doctors were contemplating feeding her through a tube placed through the nose to the stomach.

I went close to her and asked, 'You said you did not travel.' And she concurred. She was home. Then I asked her, 'By home, did you mean Kerala, your home state, or your home here in Kochi?'

She said, 'Kerala.'

My brain lit up and my heart beat faster.

'Did you travel out of Kochi, within Kerala?'

She nodded.

'Where?' I asked her.

She looked at me, tired, and said, 'Thiruvananthapuram.'

Without wasting another second, I called the ICU nurse. I asked her to start Silvia on the drug that was going to help her get out of the ICU, get her to a room, get her discharged and get her back home to her chubby little one-year-old buttercup, who was waiting for her for more than a week.

What was this miracle treatment? The antibiotic Doxycycline.

The Child of the Mother

Historically, this infection has been around for a very long time. It was first described in China in the ancient clinical text *Zhouhofang.* In 610 CE, Yuan-Fang Chao described this infection in his poem. Shi-Zhen Li, the famous Chinese physician monk, discussed the characteristics of this dreadfully difficult to diagnose disease in his book *Ben Cao Gang Mu* in 1596. More than 1,000 years ago, the Chinese called this strangely terrifying disease that sometimes killed 'sihashitsu'; it was caused by the bite of the 'sna ra', or the red mite. As medical science and our understanding of the germ theory of infectious diseases evolved, 'sihashitsu' was replaced by its current name.

Scrub typhus.

Scrub typhus is caused by the bacteria *Orientia tsutsugamushi* (belonging to the family of microbes known as Rickettsiaceae), from the Japanese 'tsutsuga' meaning illness and 'mushi' meaning bug or insect. It is spread through the bite of trombiculid mite larvae, or chiggers. Scrub typhus is a systemic illness that can present as FUO. If left untreated, it can lead to death.

India belongs to the 'tsutsugamushi triangle' (along with Pakistan, Japan and Australia), where scrub typhus accounts for at least one-fourth of FUO. A scar-like scab called the 'eschar' at the bite site is a good indicator of infection, but is not always visible or identifiable in all patients. This was explicitly missing in Silvia. The absence of definitive symptoms and signs on clinical examination, and general dependence on blood investigations make scrub typhus quite challenging to discern from other forms of fever-related illnesses. The involvement of the liver is possible, though rare. But this was important. Scrub typhus, because it mimics many different infections, with a delayed diagnosis, can kill the person and can affect any organ system, including the liver, presenting as hepatitis. A rare but important feature is the low-level jaundice but very high liver-enzyme levels, which was peculiarly notable in Silvia's case.

As scrub typhus is not commonly found everywhere, there are pockets where it is usually identified easily. One such pocket, reported extensively in news media, was Thiruvananthapuram city in Kerala, where a large number of cases and deaths due to this infection were reported.

Scrub typhus is curable if identified early. The antibiotic of choice is the tetracycline group of drugs. Doxycycline melts the little but terrifying critter like a hot knife to butter. Twenty-four hours after starting the antibiotic, Silvia began to show signs of rapid improvement and early recovery. Her appetite was coming back too. So was mine. In three days, she was shifted out of the ICU. On the eighth day, Silvia was sent home to her sweet infant, about whom she had mumbled in her sleep almost every night inside my ICU. Her father tagged along, tired but glad. He was not anxious or angry anymore.

~

That evening, I returned home to find a plate of hot, freshly fried banana fritters and a pot of steaming coffee on the table.

Outside, on my balcony, I sat down to enjoy the little snack in solitude, watching the backwater surface ripple lightly, as a gentle breeze blew over it in the distance.

I got up only after every bit of those fritters was finished, and the pot of coffee was empty.

But it was not only my stomach that was filled.

My heart and mind were full.

Filled to the brim, and exhaustingly content, I heaved a sigh of relief.
A sigh meaningful only to me.
I closed my eyes.
I was back at a familiar place.
There was a brick wall.
A rice field surrounded it.
And there was a lake.
Little spotted fish at the glistening surface.
A cool breeze.
I was going to stay there a while.

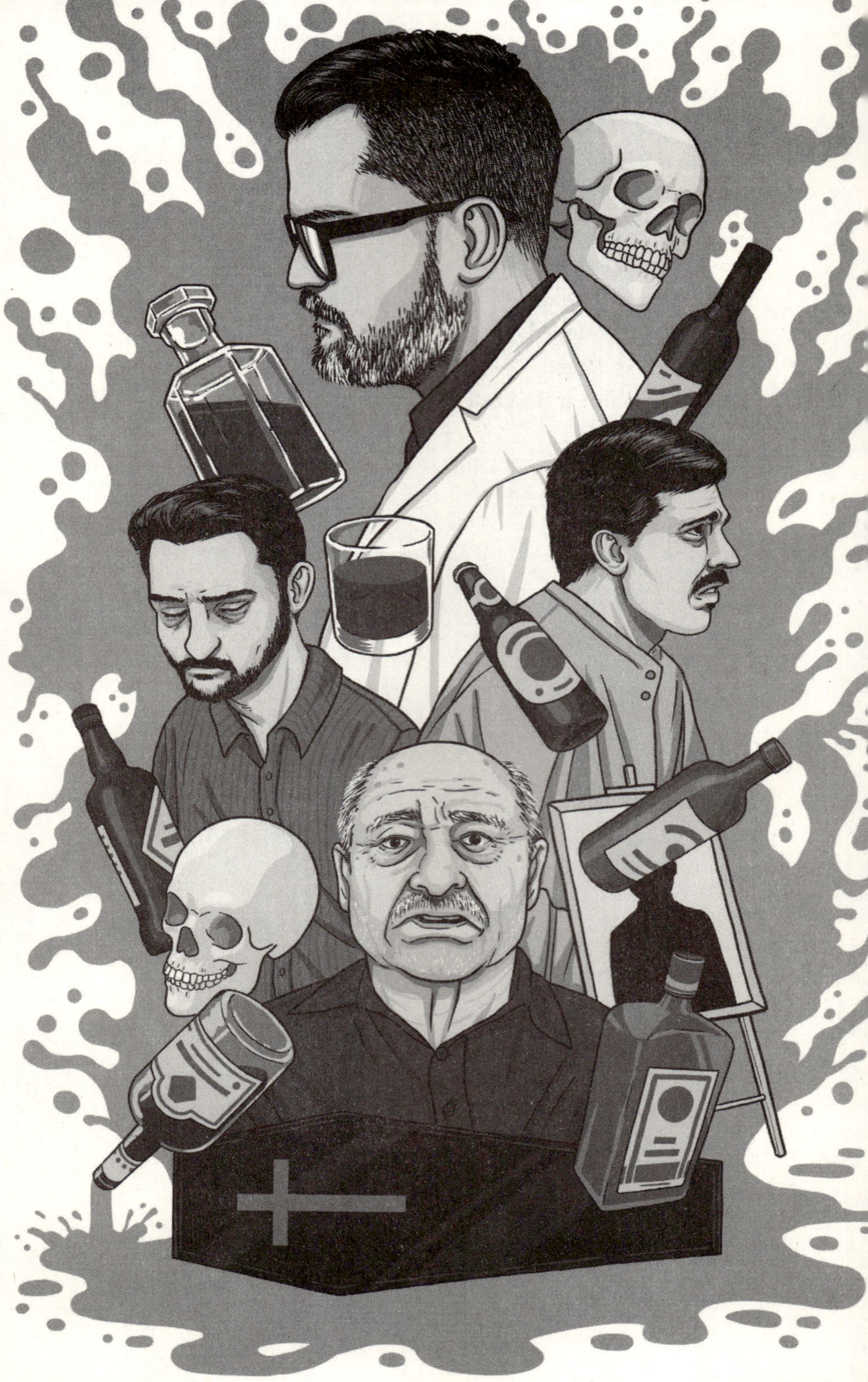

CHAPTER 6

A Miracle at the Wedding Feast at Cana

The Malady of Alcohol-Associated Liver Disease

Parasite

'Be sober-minded; be watchful. Your adversary, the devil, prowls around like a roaring lion, seeking someone to devour.'
—1 PETER 5:8, THE HOLY BIBLE

THE HORN SNAIL LIVES IN THE VAST OCEAN, BUT IT IS NOT alone. Something constantly searches for it, sensing its presence. Once found, that something begins its life—the parasitic fluke *Euhaplorchis californiensis*. This worm starts its life cycle inside the horn snail, laying eggs and producing larvae. These larvae have a singular mission: to find their next host, the aquatic killifish.

Without the fish, the larvae cannot reach their final destination—the intestines of a water bird, where they grow and reproduce. To get there, the larvae must ensure that the infected killifish is eaten by a bird. And they do, in a chillingly effective way.

The larvae attach to the killifish's gills, then invade its brain, where they release powerful chemicals. These chemicals then lower serotonin and spike dopamine levels in the fish's brain, causing it to behave erratically—shaking, jerking and swimming aggressively. These bizarre movements attract birds, who eat the fish and, unknowingly, the parasites. Inside the bird's gut, the worms mature, mate and are expelled back into the water via droppings, restarting their life cycle in another horn snail.

A similar parasite, the Gordian worm or hairworm, begins life on land but must return to water to reproduce. Its larvae infect arthropods like beetles and mantises, but its preferred host is the wood cricket. After the cricket consumes worm eggs near water, the larvae grow inside it, feeding on the host.

To reproduce, the mature worm needs water. It controls the cricket by altering its brain chemistry by reducing serotonin, boosting dopamine and crazily driving it towards light. Reflections of moonlight on water lure the cricket to jump into lakes or streams, where it drowns, allowing the worm to emerge, find a mate and begin the cycle again.

Both the killifish and the cricket lose control of their actions, becoming puppets of the parasites. All due to the chemical manipulation of their brains.

Dopamine and serotonin, though both neurotransmitters, are profoundly different. Serotonin promotes mood stability and contentment, telling the brain, 'This feels good, and I've had enough.' Its deficiency can lead to aggression or suicidal behaviour. Dopamine drives motivation and desire, saying, 'This feels good, I want more.' It often fuels addiction. Where serotonin brings peace, dopamine brings obsession—and in the hands of a parasite, total control.

Do you know something else that does the same to the human brain, exactly like these parasitic worms?

Alcohol.

It increases dopamine reward signals in the brain so much that women and men come under its control. Soon after, it gets to the breaking point, as it reduces serotonin to such an extent that true happiness seems lost, depression takes over and people become suicidal or stop feeling for the world around them. To balance out the depression, alcohol—the socially accepted poison, this parasitic substance, also known as ethanol—tells the human brain to keep depending on it to feel that reward, even when it has already driven the host deep inside a dark void. In this dark place, alcohol modifies and shows deep worries dressed in bittersweet drama. The sweetness then becomes a calling, the bitterness driving yearning for the sweetness, in a vicious cycle that the consumer can't make head or tail of. If the consumer is deprived of alcohol, its absence makes them shallow and aggressive, impulsive and regressive, driving them to death—like how the worm affects the killifish. Once they keep getting a steady supply of alcohol, the depression-reward cycles make the consumer behave like the wood cricket, steering them to their inevitable death.

Alcohol drives people towards violence and abuse, creates and worsens mental health disorders and promotes dissatisfaction. It ensures that its consumers stop prioritizing their lives and prioritize the bottom of a bottle instead. It takes away the pain, because it takes your mind away, never to return it. And make no mistake. It is always the first drop of alcohol that takes control. You will not realize it. It will direct you to it occasionally. Then more than occasionally, thereafter regularly, and then frequently—until it becomes your life. It breaks families and creates orphans. Alcohol is the silent but openly secret widow-maker. Every single drop of alcohol once inside the human body parasitizes the brain.

Every.

Single.

Drop.

Rage

More than two years ago, I met this young man, Nobin, who was in his early twenties. He was deeply jaundiced. His body was frail, mostly skin and bones, except his abdomen. It protruded painfully because it was fluid-filled. He was breathless the first time I saw him, and my team had to remove many litres of fluid from his distended abdomen for him to get better and breathe freely. He was going to die. We were sure that his father had got comfortable with the dreadful reality that he would have to bury his son.

Nobin had only his father as family—a slight but headstrong man in his late sixties. His mother died when he was young, from cancer of the breast that spread to her brain. Multiple sessions of chemotherapy and radiation kept her alive outside, but dead inside. But the few months they got with her were blessed. After his mother's death, the young man started consuming alcohol at a very early age—initially, to ease his petty troubles and, later, to ease the bigger ones. He never went to college and dabbled in small businesses with his friends, whom he called his 'partners'.

By the time he was with me in the ICU, he was all of twenty-four years old and had been diagnosed with acute-on-chronic liver failure (ACLF)—a terrifying condition, as you may recall, that was associated with my patient Harish in chapter 2. In ACLF, an already chronically damaged liver, stressed by ongoing alcohol abuse, develops severe swelling due to acute alcohol toxicity, called alcohol-associated hepatitis or AAH. Patients with AAH rapidly progress to liver failure and usually have a very short survival prognosis—close to 100 per cent of them die in six months due to multiple organ failure triggered by ongoing liver failure.

Nobin's father would be alone, and their family would cease to exist if the youngest member died. There was nothing we could do but aggressively manage the ACLF in every way we could. And we did. Nobin got better, and we took him through a de-addiction protocol. Through grit and the thought that his father would be alone and fearing the end of his bloodline, Nobin vanquished his vice—his alcohol use disorder got under control, and he got sober.

For over a year, Nobin's father would come along with him regularly and religiously for surveillance tests, and to make sure he followed my advice properly.

The young man was abstinent from alcohol for two years.

Not a single drop.

The father and son started their own business.

Nobin's father became his new friend and partner. The bonding took his mind off alcohol. Together, they ran a street food cart near their tiny home. In the local language, such a setup was called 'thattu kada', a makeshift food place. Every evening, the father–son duo would serve fresh, hot masala dosas, omelettes, spicy chutneys and parottas along with a variety of chicken-, beef- and fish-based side dishes. They started in the evening and went on late into the night. Business was good, and the locals loved them. During one follow-up visit, they invited me to have a meal one day at their street-food place.

Nobin told me they had a special dish every day—a warm rice kanji (porridge) with flavourful mixed pulses, pickles, spiced buttermilk and lip-smacking beef fry. In their opinion, it was the best in the city. I thought about finding the time to go there, but it was far, approximately 300 kilometres from my workplace. All through the treatment period, I made sure that the pill burden was kept to a minimum so that they could earn a livelihood and not waste money on unnecessary medications.

But one month later, Nobin missed his review. Neither Nobin nor his father visited me the following month. But their neighbours did. They wanted to speak with me and let me know something important. Since Nobin and his father always spoke well of me, and the whole locality knew me, even though they had not met me, they had come carrying a message. Nobin's father had died from a cardiac arrest triggered by a myocardial infarction (heart attack) three months before our scheduled review visit.

When grief hits out of the blue, without warning, without concern, the brain looks at ways to seek reward to make everything feel as if it is better.

In that moment of grief, Nobin started drinking again.

Heavily.

After two long years, he fell neck-deep back into the bittersweet struggle he had tried to forget. It was a journey measured in empty bottles that ended in my ICU—the only place it was ever going to go. Nobin completely lost his sense of self. It was utter and complete loss. Unstoppable alcohol binges followed. An alcohol binge is defined as a drinking pattern that corresponds to consuming five or more drinks in males, or four or more drinks in females, in about two hours.

On tragically glorious days, Nobin was drinking close to 1.2 litres of alcohol in a day. Just like the first day I met him in the ICU, he was admitted to the ICU department of a hospital in his hometown with a recurrence of severe AAH. He was going to meet his father and mother. He made sure that no one was going to stop him. When a drowning man tastes company that brings him back to the breathable surface, the loss of that company becomes untenable; it remains null and void, and there seems no other way to proceed than into the inevitable embrace of that void. As the void was where the company now existed, it was imperative to go there. Nobin was going. I knew it.

Nobin was on a mechanical ventilator that helped him breathe and in multiple organ failure because the liver injury this time had been dreadfully damaging. He made sure it was dreadfully damaging. The neighbours wanted to know if shifting him to my care in an ICU ambulance, with expenses borne by them, would be beneficial. The last time he was dying, he had got a second chance at life under my care. But I felt it. This time, it was different. He was going to die. It was inevitable. He had vomited around 2 litres of blood, and by the time he was put on the ventilator, he was already in a coma, and his kidneys had shut down by night. By morning, he went into cardiac arrest, and he was on multiple medications to get his blood pressure going.

He was not going to last the 300-kilometre journey.

I longed for that special hot rice kanji meal with Nobin and his father when they had invited me.

Maybe I should have made time for that.

Maybe we must all make time for the little things we tend to overlook, only to regret later, because we find more value for them in retrospect.

Nobin, my dear patient, would meet his father soon, and they would set up shop in the sanctuary where they belonged. He would embrace his mother, whom he had missed for so long.

Maybe I will visit that place one day, where once a food cart stood and two people in solitude served lovely meals to people on warm, humid evenings, which now lay empty.

Maybe.

~

Every week, I sign off death summaries of young and middle-aged men with liver failure, multiple organ failure and liver cancer due to alcohol use. Some of them drank heavily, while others consumed alcohol modestly. Some of my patients felt cheated. They drank with their friends, some of whom drank much more, but those friends remained healthy and productive while my patients were either on their deathbed or waiting for a liver transplant.

This begged the question, should one consume alcohol in moderation? Especially for its purported health benefits for the heart? The 'presumed benefits' of moderate drinking were first published in 1924 by biologist Raymond Pearl. In it, he concluded that the clinical effects of alcohol use followed a J-shaped curve, where to the left of the tipping point of the 'J' were non-drinkers who survived much less, and to the right were those who drank more than modestly and had increased death rates. So the key to increasing life was to drink 'moderately'. But why were they surviving better with modest use of alcohol and not no alcohol or heavy alcohol?

Further research found that a particular type of heart disease was reduced with alcohol use—called ischemic heart disease, which is a type of 'heart attack' in which the blood flow to the heart decreases and this affects patients who develop a poorly pumping heart.

But why was ischemic heart disease reduced with modest alcohol use? Fast forward to 2023, when a study by a group of doctors from

Massachusetts General Hospital found the reason was that alcohol promoted long-term reductions in stress signalling in the brain, leading to a happier and thus 'healthier' heart.

Remember the worms.

The dopamine. The mind control. The reward. The vicious cycle.

Interestingly, another study showed that the 'lowering of stress' was happening even at the molecular and cellular level, and was manifested by a reduced microvascular dysfunction or MVD—in which 'blood health' also improved with modest alcohol consumption.

So, all good, right?

Sorry, not really.

A major 2022 study published in *JAMA Network Open* by researchers from Massachusetts General Hospital and the Broad Institute showed the perceived favourable health benefits of modest alcohol use were because people with lower or modest consumption also had better and healthier lifestyles, such as dietary patterns and physical activity. When these were taken out of the equation, lower doses of alcohol increased heart disease risk—which went up exponentially with increasing dose and duration. More recent studies suggested that the association of low-to-moderate alcohol consumption with the reduction in cardiovascular disease risk was a result of lifestyle changes and that any reduction in alcohol consumption was, in fact, beneficial in terms of general health. Quite interestingly, in those with worse health outcomes and low or modest consumption, the genetic profile also played a role. If one did not have good genes, any amount of alcohol was going to hurt. The best way to protect yourself is not to consume alcohol at all because, even now, the 'good' genes are not yet fully identified (and probably will never be; it also does not matter in the bigger picture). So everyone is at risk of dreadful diseases from any amount of alcohol, until proven otherwise. While light or moderate drinkers lowered their risk for ischemic heart disease, the 2023 Massachusetts General Hospital study also showed that any amount of alcohol increased the risk of various cancers and hence increased chances of cancer-related death, even when the person had a 'supposedly healthy heart'. This was again proven in a monumental study by researchers from Canada and the United Kingdom, published in 2023, which showed that low-volume alcohol drinking was not associated with protection against death from any cause and that it, in fact, increased risk of death, more in women than men.

But then people who supported the alcohol lobby came with all sorts of studies by playing a great deal of mental gymnastics. One study showed that people with modest alcohol use gained one whole year in their lifetime! However, the gain of one year by modest drinkers was offset by a twofold to fourfold increase in mouth (oral) and food-pipe (oesophageal) cancers, and drinking beyond a modest amount led to a significant loss of life expectancy. To top it off, like placing a rotten black cherry on top of alcohol connoisseurs' happy but stale cake, scientists again proved that any level of alcohol was unsafe because it increased the risk of various other types of cancers far too significantly. After all, alcohol is inherently a DNA-damaging poison—a carcinogen.

The verdict is in: There is *no* safe level of alcohol that benefits human health.

Alcohol controls the brain every single time we allow it to. When used at regular intervals, we rent out our brains—and, in the long term, our lives—to its calling.

I rage inside, wishing everyone, young and old, man, woman and child, knew this.

Regret

A patient's wife walked into my outpatient department on a warm, sunny afternoon in April 2023. She handed me a small plastic packet. It contained three laddus. It was her husband Paul's birthday.

The wife told me she was happy and that the family was doing good for themselves.

I looked around for Paul.

~

My patient, Paul, suffered from alcohol use disorder. He had been drinking for more than fifteen years. Three months ago, he developed severe alcohol-related hepatitis. Jaundiced, with a massively distended abdomen due to complicated fluid collection, battling a severe bacterial infection of the blood and disoriented due to brain failure and in extreme liver failure, he was transferred to our clinical unit for expert care, optimization and the possibility of a liver transplant to help him survive. Unfortunately, liver transplantation was not an option from the outset.

Paul owned a small provisions and bakery shop, had two daughters (aged five and nine) and his wife, Celine, had worked part-time doing errands but quit her job after the girls were born. They did not have enough money to evaluate Paul for the transplant. Without the option of curative surgery, Paul was put on the best medical-care support we could provide him. Antibiotics, human albumin infusions, specialized treatments at a fraction of the cost and nutritional therapy became cornerstones of his care.

Miraculously, he responded to it. To everyone's surprise and glee.

Paul's alcohol-related hepatitis resolved, and he went back to being a stable cirrhosis patient, away from the life-and-death situation he had put himself into. We put him on a psychiatric programme to prevent relapse. He did well for three months. Then he stopped coming to my outpatient department and started missing his surveillance tests and de-addiction protocol reviews.

Like clockwork, Paul relapsed. Initially, to 200 ml per day, and then to almost a litre of alcohol daily. Paul's cousins dragged him to my outpatient department one day, and I got to know of his terrible relapse.

He had stopped his medications and was back with his 'good company'. He even paid for everyone's drinks. He sometimes abused and harassed Celine to forcefully take away money from the shop. In his absence, she tried to run the shop to put food into their children's stomachs and pay for their school tuition fees. Paul sometimes beat Celine in front of their children. The days were chaotic, and life dimly lit. There was no hope.

I spoke to Paul and told him that it was a disease. That it was not his fault, and that he needed help. That his friends were not real friends, and that his daughters needed their father. He cried a lot in front of me, in front of his wife and the children, in my outpatient room, and told me that alcohol was a more attractive option than anything else. It was his life. He was in too deep. He wanted to stop in words, but he could not. He could not because, deep inside, he did not want to. He wanted to get away from his life. Alcohol made him find life in death. After much ado, he agreed to enter de-addiction and went back into the protocol, but then also went back to drinking. Hospital visits, medicine expenses and the costs of buying alcohol for himself and his friends became a worryingly big deal. He started borrowing. Debts were rising.

One day, Celine came into my outpatient alone and asked me to stop getting Paul better.

'Let him remain sick,' she told me. 'If he gets better, he goes back to drinking and we lose money. Let him remain sick so we can earn enough from the store to get through. He will remain home, and I can work at the shop and provide for us all.'

She was serious.

A couple of months later, after an eventful episode of binge drinking, Paul developed a severe complication of his underlying liver disease. It was far worse than the first time I had seen him during the referral to our ICU. The severe alcohol-related hepatitis was back. His kidneys were injured. The family denied admission. They had no money to spare. It would have to come from the daughters' education fund that Celine had kept aside. They lived very far away. Almost 400 kilometres from where I worked.

I told them that I would be happy to refer him to a public hospital for comfort care. Celine took Paul home.

For the next two weeks, I regularly prescribed medications, made suggestions to reduce symptoms and comforted the family over the phone while Paul was treated at his home. A good physician nearby would administer antibiotics and fluids to Paul as he got sicker and closer to death.

Paul died at home on the eighteenth day after I diagnosed him with a recurrent episode of severe alcohol-related hepatitis that progressed to multiple organ failure.

Three months after his death, Celine came to visit me from their faraway home on Paul's birthday to give me sweets. Three laddus. One from her and the other two from their two daughters.

Because I never stigmatized her or Paul.

I did not make her look like a failure.

I never blamed Paul for his behaviour.

They were free now. The girls went to school and Celine was running the shop well.

But all I could think about was that fourth laddu.

The one I never received from Paul because he died.

A woman lost her husband, two young girls lost their father, and I lost a patient who had etched himself into my heart—into a scar I now carry. Three lives shattered, and nothing could ever fill that void. I never recommend alcohol, not even in moderation, because I carry the trauma of watching families being torn apart by it. That day, as I rode home, hidden from my driver's gaze, I ate three small laddus in silence at the back of my car. The sweetness that filled my mouth, unable to cloak the heaviness in my chest. I fell asleep mid-journey, only to be awakened at my doorstep, still lost in thoughts of life, death and the helplessness in between.

In some moments, I feel less like a doctor and more like a ferryman—caught between struggling to save lives and witnessing them slip away. Medicine stops being just science; it becomes service. I begin to understand that, often, no pill can match the power of a comforting word, a quiet presence or a gentle touch. Even when nothing more can be done clinically, offering hope—however fragile, through empathy and human connection—gives my role meaning. And in that, I find purpose.

Like that time when the friends of my patient, Latheef, a thirty-three-year-old man, came to me to convey the message that he had died by suicide. On the way to Kasargod town, he jumped onto the tracks from the moving train and was crushed and dismembered to death. Latheef had been suffering from alcohol use disorder and had barely survived a severe episode of alcohol-related hepatitis a while back.

The new viral pandemic had destroyed Latheef's travel and photography business. He could never recover the losses. It was as if he decided he wanted to die because he could hardly provide for his family, and had become dependent on his elderly parents.

It took me and my team a whole lot of shouldering burdens to get him out of the ICU and send him home. He went through a de-addiction protocol and was off alcohol for two months. But on that train, he had been partly inebriated. He left behind his wife, aged twenty-nine, and a cherub of a three-year-old daughter.

People often cling to the idea of an afterlife where spirits linger out of love, but that's grief creating comfort where there is none. When someone dies, they cease to exist—just as they did before birth. They become memories for the living to grow around and eventually forget. This is why I'm overwhelmed when a patient dies—not because they're somewhere else, but because they're simply gone, forever. The real value lies in living, not in romanticizing death. Alcohol hastens that end, like the killifish and cricket controlled by parasites—stripping away reason while offering an illusion of peace. Even the best doctors' advice and care cannot compete with what patients believe lies at the bottom of a bottle.

Alcohol's damage goes far beyond the liver. It is the brain that pays the heaviest price. It shrinks brain volume, erodes grey matter, impairs memory formation, slows processing and blunts emotional awareness—making it impossible to recognize the consequences of one's actions. It feeds anxiety and depression, worsens psychiatric conditions and disrupts sleep. Every drink offers a dopamine hit, a lie dressed as reward, pushing people further into dependence. You never know when alcohol will strike or how deeply it will ruin you. If alcohol is your friend, you don't need enemies.

Redemption

During one routine day on ward rounds, I received a call from the emergency department for a consult on a patient referred for our expert opinion, further care and treatment, if the family was willing to be admitted.

'They are willing to get admitted,' said my emergency physician. 'They have nowhere to go. The family says the patient has been given three months to live. They want to try this place as a last resort, but the family has made its decision and is willing to carry his lifeless body away if nothing works out.'

His wife was desperate. His time was running out.

'What did they say he has?' I asked her.

'Severe alcoholic hepatitis,' she told me.

And I thought to myself, *This is true. The doctors are right. The diagnosis meant he had very little time to live.*

The patient was a middle-aged man called James. He was quite sick, deeply jaundiced, confused and incoherent. James had been using alcohol daily for the past eight years. For the past two years, he had started drinking excessively, and he almost always drank alone. He woke up only to start drinking and would complete at least a litre of alcohol by the end of the day. He ate very little. When alcohol took over, his primary necessities took a back seat. The drink, its odour, that bitter feeling inside his mouth and that final spark at the end of the drink—it was dominating him, like an inescapable seductress.

People do not enjoy alcohol. Alcohol enjoys the people who consume it, as it feeds on their rationality, integrity, logic and thought. Beyond a certain point, people unknowingly rent their brains out to alcohol. James had crossed that point many years ago. His last alcohol use was three days before the current onset of jaundice. He was obese and without other chronic ailments. The Covid-19 pandemic affected his work. His travel business suffered, and he had to sell most of his vehicles. This was important to note because the pandemic drove increased alcohol use around the world—a silent pandemic inside a pandemic that no one talked about. One month before, James's friends noticed that his eyes were yellow, and that he drank less than he used to. He lacked appetite, and his sleep was extremely disturbed.

He was taken to a nearby clinic, where they found that his bilirubin level was high. After much persuasion, James met a gastroenterologist for further evaluation and management. At the hospital, he was thoroughly evaluated for all causes of jaundice, and more importantly, doctors assessed if his alcohol use was 'significant' enough to cause alcohol-related liver disease. To assess this, a scoring system was used, the Alcohol Use Disorders Identification Test-Consumption, or the AUDIT-C. If the patient had a score above 5, it meant that they had significant alcohol use, and if the score was more than 10, it meant they were alcohol dependent. James's score was 11, which was highly suggestive of alcohol dependence. Tests for viral hepatitis and autoimmune liver disease, chronic infections affecting the liver, rare genetic liver diseases (such as Wilson's disease) and iron-overload conditions affecting the liver (called hemochromatosis) came back negative. The provisional diagnosis at the first hospital was severe AAH. However, certain boxes had to be ticked to fulfil the diagnosis of AAH, using specific criteria.

The National Institute on Alcohol Abuse and Alcoholism devised the criteria wherein if the clinical and blood test criteria were met and a liver biopsy was compatible with severe alcohol-related liver injury, then the diagnosis of AAH was definite. However, if the liver-biopsy testing expertise were unavailable, a score equivalent to 'probable AAH' was good enough to diagnose the condition for further treatment consideration.

The first medical centre James was admitted to did not have the availability of liver-biopsy services. It was not a simple liver biopsy (in which a needle is inserted into the liver under ultrasound scan guidance across the skin) that James required. He required a special type of biopsy called transjugular liver biopsy (the history of which is described in the prologue)—in which a wire and a needle are guided through a blood vessel in the neck into the liver, and a piece of liver tissue is retrieved and removed through a sheath placed within the large neck vein. This specialized form of liver biopsy is done when patients suffer from severe liver disease with a high risk of bleeding and fluid accumulation in the abdomen. Since James was also obese, we had to be sure that the severe hepatitis was due to alcohol per se and not due to non-alcohol-related fatty deposits and related inflammation in the presence of his underlying morbid obesity. Another scoring system was used to assess this. In the Alcoholic Liver Disease/Non-alcoholic Fatty Liver Index, or ANI, in short, James had a score above 20, which effectively meant that the reason for his severe liver disease was, in all probability, related to alcohol use.

In those patients who do not disclose significant alcohol use, there are other ways to get the truth out of them when a liver biopsy cannot be performed or consent for the same is not received. People lie, but their blood does not. A series of blood tests can identify when a person consumed alcohol, as well as how much. This is known as the phosphatidyl ethanol or PEth test. The level of PEth in the blood is helpful in identifying alcohol use behaviour in the patient. A PEth value of less than 10 μg/L indicates that the patient was abstinent or that it is improbable that alcohol consumption has occurred. PEth values from 35–210 μg/L means that the person is a social drinker, and >210 μg/L is suggestive of excessive alcohol use. When PEth tests are not available, toxicologists resort to looking directly at alcohol level in the most commonly accessible sampling sites—urine, if the drink was within three days; blood, if it was within three weeks; and nails and hair, if the alcohol use was suspected to be within three months. In James, the significant alcohol use from clinical history, the exclusion of other causes for jaundice, and specific scores strongly suggestive of alcohol dependence precluded the need for specialized tests to quantify and confirm alcohol in his body.

Now that doctors had a diagnosis of probable AAH, they wanted to ensure that it was a severe form of the disease, since only severe forms require active drug treatments because they are associated with worse clinical outcomes. The mild form does not require treatment but only supportive care and abstinence. In severe forms of AAH, without response to standard care medications, patients have a high risk of dying without timely liver transplantation. Various scores are used to diagnose severe AAH. The Model for End-Stage Liver Disease (MELD) score and Maddrey's (MDF) are the most used. A patient with MELD ≥21 or an MDF ≥32 is considered to have a severe form of AAH, and requires immediate drug therapy to reduce liver disease severity. In James, the MELD was 30 and the MDF was 98.6—which meant that without treatment, his chance of dying at one month was 65 per cent.

Treatment of severe AAH was introduced correctly only in 1978 by Professor Willis Maddrey, who also discovered the MDF score. Currently a wise eighty-year-old professor at the University of Texas Southwestern Medical Center, his work on the use of steroids for the treatment of severe AAH was a game-changer. Even though it did not impact long-term survival, short-term survival was vastly improved with steroid therapy. His original study, done decades before, is still considered and recommended as the first-line treatment for severe AAH. But there was more to it. The response to steroids was determined to be far more important than just the treatment initiation.

In 2007, researchers at the Hôpital Claude Huriez in Lille, France, developed a score to identify patients who would respond to steroids, called the Lille Model. If the Lille score was <0.45, then the patient was considered to have a complete response to steroid treatment and the entire twenty-eight-day treatment course of steroids was completed. However, if the score was >0.45, then the patient was considered a non-responder to treatment and was further managed only with supportive care or offered a liver transplantation. In most cases, without a timely liver transplant, almost all patients died even on best supportive care. As per the rule of the book, James was started on steroids, and his Lille score was scrutinized at the end of seven days. Unfortunately, his score was 0.48—which meant that he was a non-responder and there was no benefit in treating him further with steroids.

But there was still a ray of hope deep within the published medical literature. In 2011, the same researchers from Lille had found three types of responders to steroids, with response scores sub-divided into <0.16, the complete responder; >0.16 but <0.56, the partial responder; and >0.56, the original non-responder. This meant that James was a partial responder to steroids. Partial responders had three options. Continue steroids only for the full twenty-eight days and hope for the best, or add a drug called N-acetylcysteine or another called metadoxine to improve steroid response. The doctors added N-acetylcysteine to the drug treatment for James, hoping that his jaundice would resolve. But after twenty-eight days of treatment, his jaundice level shot up from 5.5 mg/dl to 32 mg/dl. James became disoriented with the development of hepatic encephalopathy, due to the progression of his liver failure, and was in grave danger of going into a liver coma (the last stage of hepatic encephalopathy) and dying within three months, as predicted. With no other option other than liver transplantation, James was referred to our unit for further management.

The challenge with liver transplantation after the diagnosis of severe AAH is that since patients like James were recent alcohol users, they lacked the insight to understand the seriousness of the realistic harms of alcohol use even after a life-saving liver transplant surgery. This means that the chance of such patients relapsing on alcohol after liver transplantation is relatively high. They are likely to have a false sense of security that with a new liver in place, everything will be fine. In such a scenario, doctors generally consider a six-month sobriety period for ideally transplanting such patients. But James did not have six months. He was going to die in three.

However, bringing new hope, novel studies showed that transplanting patients with severe AAH quite early, disregarding the sobriety period, also gave good clinical outcomes and lower relapse rates—provided it was done through a unique screening protocol and waitlist times for receiving an organ on time were not challenging. But this was all good in the West, where transplantation was part of universal health coverage and livers from cadavers or brain-dead donors were readily available. But in James's case, it was different. The family did not have a donor, and they did not even have enough money to work up a donor to assess suitability. They had a young daughter who was in school and no one else. The financial crisis was looming above their heads.

When there is surety that the patient will die, physicians start looking at all things medical in black and white. Either they throw everything at the patient as part of an 'aggressive' and upgraded treatment, including medications and procedures that are not effectively evidence-based, or they comfort the family and take patients on their final journey with dignity.

Death is the bigger business for corporate hospitals.

This was true for patients like James, who, as per medical science, were sure not to make it. However, the family was not willing to let go. That little sliver of hope was always the milking point for corporate greed. Treating hospitals would stop serving the best interests of the patient, but start serving those of the family members, leading to a vicious cycle of monetary loss that paralleled the inevitable loss of life. Moreover, families would be run into the ground, in poverty, with just a medical bill along with a death certificate.

But then there was also a third group of physicians who believed that the art and heart of clinical medicine practice was not to let go but to hold on rationally, driven by reason and logic.

So my team and I started to think about doing things that were not conventionally done, but would not be a financial strain on the family either.

We closed all textbooks and protocols.

We shut down the routine algorithmic management.

We cleaned the slate and started afresh.

A life is priceless, and saving one is never left to chance but to relentless persistence. In medicine, offering comfort to the dying and hope to the hopeless demands not just skill, but deep humanism. It often costs us sleep, appetite and mental peace. James didn't choose alcohol use disorder; it was a disease born from broken hope and harsh circumstance. Like many others, he too would have wanted a second chance—and everyone, even at their worst, deserves one. For me and my team, nothing mattered more than the patient and their family, and James became our singular focus. As Paracelsus said, 'The art of medicine has its roots in the heart.' That belief led me, one solemn evening, to search deep inside history itself for a way to save him.

~

Three thousand years ago, traditional Chinese medicine practitioners mentioned something strange in their first book on prescriptions. The use of human faeces as a 'drug'.

Fast forward to the Han and Jin dynasty periods in ancient China. Monk physicians were collecting fresh faeces from healthy children, then diluting them to make 'yellow soup' to treat sick children with severe diarrhoeal disease and infections of the stomach and intestines. In the late seventeenth century, veterinarians treated sick horses and cattle by giving them faeces from healthy animals. Not until 1958 did we have documented evidence of what was happening with this strange therapy, in which the sick were being fed faecal matter to cure certain diseases.

A surgeon, Ben Eiseman, saw that after surgery many patients were dying due to a severe diarrhoeal disease known at the time as pseudomembranous colitis. This disease was later called *Clostridioides difficile* infection. Dr Eiseman did something different. He made enemas out of fresh faeces from healthy volunteers and packed them into the rectums of patients who were sick with *C. difficile* infection. To his surprise, all of them improved, and their diarrhoeal disease ceased. Years later, clinical researchers in the Netherlands tested Eiseman's pilot study with more attentiveness and in a far better controlled environment. They found that healthy donor stool transplantation, where faecal suspensions from healthy persons were infused into the intestines, technically known as FMT or faecal microbiota transplantation, cured patients with recurrent *C. difficile* infection. The US Food and Drug Administration approved FMT as the recommended treatment for patients with severe recurrent infections due to *C. difficile*.

But then something intriguing happened in the field of liver diseases. Dr Martha Llopis from France found that there were drastic changes within the bacterial population inside the gut of mice who were fed alcohol. They found that in the presence of alcohol, 'bad' bacteria emerged in the gut of these rodents while the 'good' bacteria were 'forcefully' reduced—resulting in harmful bacterial products that attacked the liver and gave rise to severe alcohol-related hepatitis-like illness in mice. Around the same time, another scientist, Dr Gladys Ferrere, also from France, found that manipulating and 'forcing' the 'bad' bacteria in mice into becoming 'good' using faeces from healthy rodents reduced alcohol-related liver injury in the small animals significantly. Stool transplantation in mice was easy to perform because mice and rats are coprophagic—meaning that they love to eat their own or another rodent's faeces. When mice with sick livers due to alcohol consumption consumed the stool of healthy mice when they were housed together, not only did their liver functions get better, but further injury from additional alcohol use was also prevented.

This evidence from animal experiments was good enough for me to consider something analogous in humans. From 2014 to 2015, as part of my thesis work, my working group at the Institute of Liver and

Biliary Sciences, New Delhi, performed the first stool transplant series in patients with severe alcohol-associated hepatitis who were not ideal candidates for liver transplantation, were not fit enough for steroid therapy and had failed to improve with standard medical care. In short, these were patients who were going to die anyway, with any level of desperate medical measures we threw at them. But what I found was surprising. Almost 90 per cent of patients who were supposed to die but received FMT survived up to one year, compared to only one-third of patients who survived after receiving only standard medical care and not FMT. This gave such patients, without any realistic medical care, a new chance at life. It did not end there.

Years later, when we looked at the sickest severe alcohol-associated hepatitis group of patients—that is, those with ACLF who had a 100 per cent risk of dying at six months—the use of FMT from healthy stool donors improved survival in up to 58 per cent for more than one and a half years.

And here was James, the sickest of the lot, his wife and child waiting for the husband, the father, to get a second chance at life. In a confused but not yet comatose James, we placed a feeding tube through the nose into the small intestine under X-ray guidance. We gave him freshly processed healthy donor stool suspension, 100 ml daily, for seven days. James spent the next twelve days in the ICU while we waited for a trillion little good guys, now inside, to do their work on him. When a high load of good bacteria enters the intestines, it replaces and overwhelms the bad ones and their damaging functions (that attack the person's liver) and restore healthy balance to the gut. Twelve days whooshed by, and every day, slowly and steadily, James became more wakeful, spoke better, and his jaundice (reflected by the bilirubin level on blood tests) started to show a downward trend.

This was it.

The little guys were doing the considerable work. With the harmful bacteria getting hit from all sides, good products from the beneficial bacteria were helping the liver and stabilizing the forgiving organ's function.

After two whole weeks, James was shifted to the room, and after a week, his bilirubin levels were 10 mg/dl, down from the previously dreadful 32 mg/dl. He was discharged home with his wife and daughter flanking his sides, hand in hand.

James had come almost comatose to us, on a bed, and walked back home with his family. Before they left, his wife thanked me and the team for an outcome they considered a miracle. Ironically, I remembered that Jesus's first miracle, the changing of water to wine, was on his mother's advice.

'This is not a miracle,' I told her. 'It is called medical science.'

I asked James if he would ever go back to drinking again, because I was left with no options or material for further 'miracles'.

And he confidently said, 'No.'

He meant it, and I knew it, even though I did refer him to a de-addiction programme later.

After all, big surprises come in small packages.

Requiem

'Could I have a prescription for some painkillers?' the mild-mannered woman asked me.

'Painkillers are not recommended for patients with cirrhosis,' I told her.

She looked unsure.

'They can cause kidney injury. Best to use the safest one, paracetamol,' I assured her.

'No, sir, they are not for my husband. I want them for myself.'

I remember this woman, even after so many years. I remember her face. She looked so tired. Her body pained. Every inch of it. Her husband beat her every single day after he got drunk; he stopped beating her only after he got so intoxicated that he either passed out on the balcony outside or inside the small office of their home. The longest he did not beat her was a month, when he was admitted with severe complications from liver disease. Hardly a month. Half the time, he was in a coma in the ICU due to severe alcohol-related liver disease; and the other half, he was being rehabilitated for discharge back home.

They did not have children.

And now, here she was, standing in front of me.

Her hands were clutched together like she was praying.

~

'Do you remember us?' she asked me.

It had been almost twelve months. Her husband, Nigil, was with her. He looked well. Nigil was one of the recipients of a stool transplant on a case basis because the family did not have the money or potential liver donors for a curative transplant when he was critically ill. After the stool transplant that saved his life, he stopped drinking. He went cold turkey. He did not even require an entry into a de-addiction programme. They were so happy. He was back working, and she never felt those bodily pains again.

Nigil was one of many.

James's story was similar to Nigil's. James quit alcohol and never relapsed.

When these cases of alcohol abstinence in the absence of drug therapy for de-addiction started popping up in the long term, I was astonished, curious and confused—all at the same time.

But there were answers.

All these people had one thing in common.

At some point during their treatment period with me, I offered a requiem for them in my heart and mind. A dirge for the repose of the dead. They were all dead men to start with because of the severe alcohol-related liver disease that afflicted them. But then the other commonality shone through. They received FMT, and my requiem was meaningless, to my great relief.

But the question lingered: Why did these men quit drinking when they were not explicitly treated for their addiction? And I found my answers emerging in the form of surprising evidence from the lab bench to the hospital bedside, from studies on mice and men.

There is something we all need to know about mice in general. They love alcohol, just like humans. They drink more alcohol than other small experimental animals and consume it like humans. If you give mice the option of alcohol compared to other options for a drink, they will choose the alcohol in the blink of an eye, and sometimes binge it too.

Let me tell you about a study and why it mattered.

There was a group of mice bred explicitly by humans for experimentation. They were called germ-free mice, which means that they lack all microbes in their bodies and are housed in tightly controlled, sterile and monitored isolation chambers to prevent contamination. This meant that they will only have the microbe(s) scientists put inside them. In effect, if the scientists put a single species of bacteria in germ-free mice, they will harbour only that bacterial species, and one could study how that group of bacteria would affect the animal. A group of researchers collected stool from people who experienced a reduced craving for alcohol after a healthy donor stool transplant, and fed the stool to a group of germ-free mice. They took another group and fed them sterile liquid—a solution without any microbes in it—and then put these two groups of mice in separate cages. After that, the scientists kept bowls of tap water mixed with 20 per cent alcohol in their cages. Ideally, they expected all the mice to gulp down that alcohol–water mix. But this was not what they observed. One group of mice went straight for the alcohol–water mix, while the other group did not. Curiously, the group that did not consume the alcohol–water were the ones who had received stool from humans. Meanwhile, the other group of mice, fed sterile solution instead of the stool, were happily enjoying the alcohol-infused tap water. The scientists found a reason for this. They analysed the bacterial species between groups and found that the good species belonging to the Ruminococcaceae family, which reduced the craving for alcohol in humans, were transmitted to germ-free mice through stool transplantation. The bacterial products and their functions changed the way the brains of the mice worked, causing them to lose interest in alcohol and reject it.

The same group of scientists demonstrated similar effects in humans. Stool transplants from healthy teetotallers, rich in specific groups of bacteria belonging to the families Lachnospiraceae and Ruminococcaceae, reduced the craving for alcohol in humans with alcohol use disorder. We found the same in our group of patients and in the long term. Alcohol relapse was lower (28.6 per cent) in those exposed to stool transplantation compared to those on only standard of care (53.8 per cent). The deep reasoning behind such a finding was clarified further. Bacteria in healthy stools, through the production of a compound called short-chain fatty acids, modify a unique signalling pathway in the brain called the tryptophan-kynurenine pathway, thereby reducing craving effects towards alcohol. Not just de-addiction programmes, but the little guys in us—in the form of healthy gut bacteria—could help battle bigger demons with the potential to control our minds in the context of alcohol dependency. As science progresses, we may unlock much more power from such bacteria. Maybe someday, but not in my lifetime, there will be a time when doctors will not have to silently include a requiem for their patients during the treatment of dreadful diseases such as severe alcohol-associated hepatitis.

In my outpatient practice, the largest group of seriously ill patients I see are those with alcohol-related liver disease. Managing such cases, especially when advanced, is the ultimate test of a physician's knowledge, judgement and empathy. Sadly, I've often seen patients with alcohol use disorder abandoned by senior doctors who deemed them 'gone cases', a label steeped in stigma. The judgement within the medical community towards these patients can be so harsh, it's sickening.

I remember one family vividly—three daughters who came to see me after their father had passed. He'd been under my care for over a year on comfort treatment, unable to afford a liver transplant. Instead, he insisted on saving his money for his youngest daughter's education. He lived far longer than expected and died peacefully at home, surrounded by his girls. When they visited, I braced for blame but was met with tears of gratitude. They told me I was the only doctor who never called their father 'an alcoholic' or blamed their mother—a cruelty they had experienced too often. One renowned gastroenterologist had even told them their father was 'just reaping what he sowed'. That kind of dehumanization still haunts me.

To me, being a doctor is not just about prescribing or trying to save every life. It's about walking with patients and families through the disease with dignity and compassion. Clinical medicine must be about treating with care, not just treatment.

Over time, I learnt that the strongest influence I could wield in alcohol de-addiction wasn't statistics or scare tactics—it was daughters. During counselling, I always asked about the patient's family, especially children. If nothing else worked, I used the 'daughter card', urging them to think about her future—her wedding, her milestones, her life without a father. I painted the painful image of a bereaved wife and a lonely daughter stepping into a future without him. I'd ask if that was really the legacy he wanted to leave behind—someone found at the bottom of a bottle?

I asked this exact question to a forty-eight-year-old patient of mine in 2023 because he was frequently relapsing on alcohol. He used to hide alcohol bottles inside the toilet flush tank of multiple bathrooms in his house, and would manage to to finish a whole bottle before bedtime without anyone noticing. I asked him to choose between 'the alcohol' or his 'two daughters', aged six and eleven. To my disheartening surprise, without any hesitation, but teary-eyed, he had most convincingly answered me, 'Alcohol.' He said he could not live without it because it swept him away from a rather dull and bitter reality, which he did not want to be a part of. He refused to see a psychiatrist, and even when he did, he refused follow-up and was adamant that he would not come for surveillance reviews. I cannot forget the bewilderment on his wife's face that day.

A few weeks later, she messaged me on my phone, thanking me for my efforts because no one, not one physician, had spent so much time trying to fight for her family and the man. I never shouted at him, made him feel bad or stigmatized him. He never felt cornered. I never made the wife feel like a failure. She was thankful for that, even though it was such hard work. Her message on my phone ended with these statements: 'He died at home yesterday early morning, after heavily drinking the previous night. He died, losing his breath, aspirating on his fresh blood vomitus in front of his children. We did not have money to take him to an ICU, and he had already stopped breathing so quickly.'

I read that last message a few times, repeatedly, and then deleted it.

Caring for people with alcohol-use disorder and their families is the most challenging of all games I am constantly playing in this bigger game called clinical medicine.

Alcohol is a recurring foe that never changes its agenda. The closest ally of my friend, Death.

As F. Scott Fitzgerald stated, 'First you take a drink, then the drink takes a drink, then the drink takes you.'

This is a hill I am willing to die on.

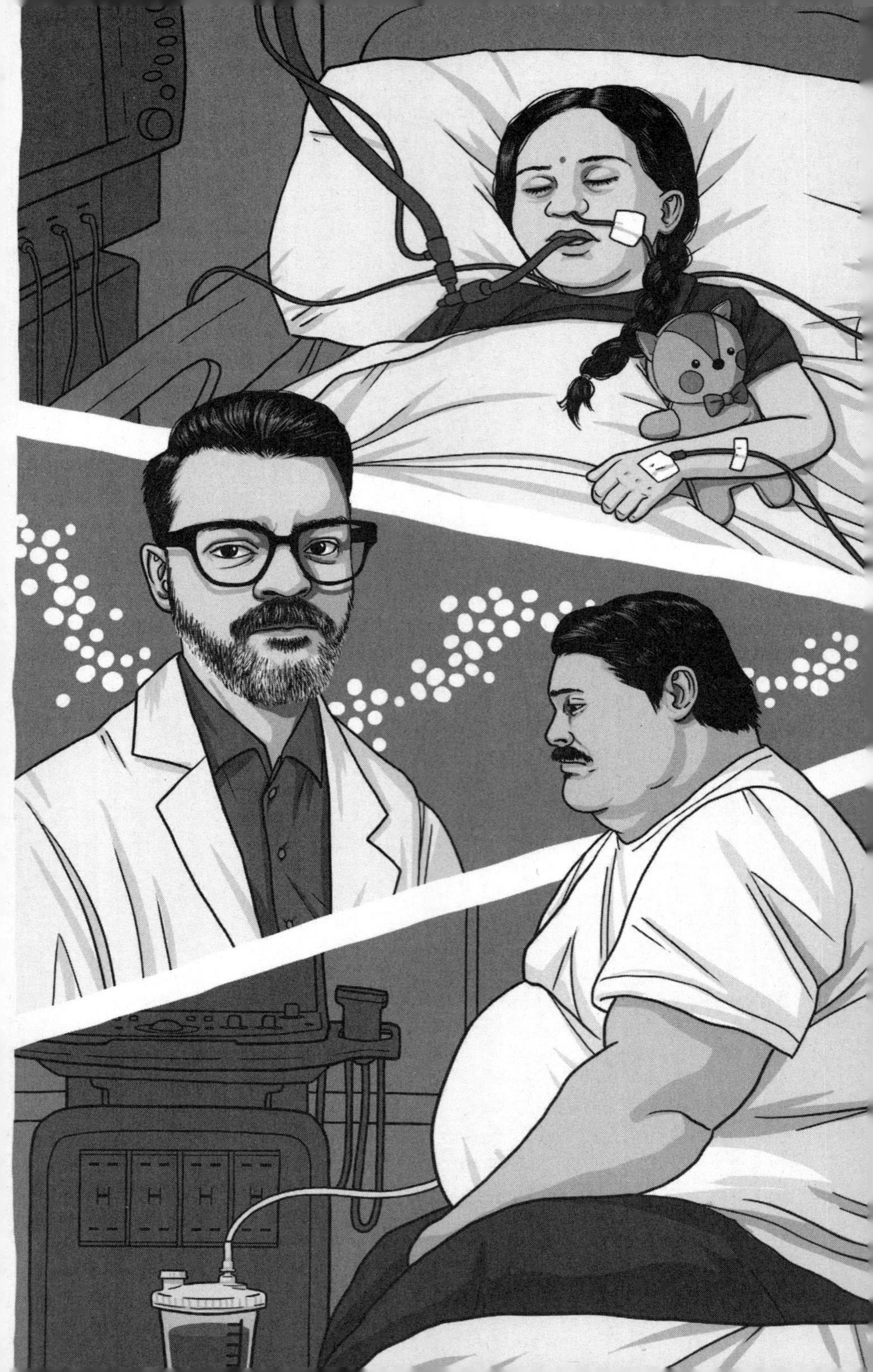

CHAPTER 7

Portrait of the Gentleman Tuscan General

Causes and Considerations in Fatty Liver Disease

The Child, Home and Hell

'The death of a child is the greatest reason to doubt the existence of God.'

—FYODOR DOSTOEVSKY

Inferno

On the day of discharge, as I was saying goodbye to a new patient in the outpatient department, Ramesh and his son came in. I stood up and shook their hands.

Ramesh gripped my left elbow and stared at me, saying nothing. But I understood the passing thoughts that lit up inside his brain and smiled at him, to which he responded, 'Thank you, sir.'

The phone rang as I saw them leave the door, and I returned to my seat. It was from the emergency room. I heard words from the other end and became concerned, as the on-call doctor spoke frantically. I had the impression that a dark cloud was hovering above me. Something sinister was on its way.

'What is it?' I inquired.

'Could you please get to the emergency room as soon as possible?' he asked hastily.

'Is the patient deeply ill?'

'Yes, and it is a little girl. Not jaundiced but appears unstable. Please come quickly,' the emergency physician hurried me, his words stumbling . . .

Before he could finish the sentence, I hung up and rushed out of the door, taking the steps down to the emergency department, unsure of the sinister battle ahead.

'THIS CHILD WAS SHIFTED FROM A HOSPITAL ABROAD,' MY emergency physician told me. The little girl had rapidly progressive hepatitis and signs of poor response.

My palms were sweaty, and my heart raced as I prepared myself to enter the medical equivalent of Dante's innermost circle of Hell: paediatric hepatology.

A week back, this chirpy little girl, Jiya, had been the happiest. Being one of the twin girls her parents cherished, she was always in the company of her sister. They were like a pair that could not be separated. Then Jiya's appetite went down the drain and her favourite foods failed to elicit excitement in her. She was not bubbly and showed less interest in playing with her twin sister. This was a big red flag because they were inseparable and constantly with each other, never a moment apart. She wanted to lie down most of the time and sleep. The next day, she developed a high-grade fever. It touched 103°F (39.4°C) and would only come down with medications and cold sponging. A day after that, the fever fluctuated, but never went away, and the child became more lethargic. The parents rushed her to a nearby clinic, where the doctor told them it was probably the seasonal flu. The doctor prescribed a short course of paracetamol for her fever, and advised the parents to keep the child well hydrated and to help her eat whatever she could, however they could. When the fever persisted, paracetamol took care of it until the following evening and then it completely disappeared. Jiya's parents were relieved, but the child was not showing any improvement in appetite or activity.

Then came the vomiting without warning. Multiple bouts of vomiting, and the child was eating and drinking much less than she was bringing out. She was getting dehydrated. This time, her parents rushed her to another hospital, a bigger one, where she was admitted to the emergency department.

'It is possibly the stomach flu,' the doctors at the new hospital assured the parents. However, the classic features of Norovirus, which was commonly responsible for the stomach flu in children and rarely in adults, were missing in her. In any case, since the treatment was only supportive care with good intravenous hydration, the doctors put Jiya on fluids and waited for her to improve. But Jiya threw new clinical challenges at them. On the fourth day, she started having severe bouts of coughing that ended with violent vomiting almost every time. Hydration efforts and anti-vomiting drugs (called anti-emetics) comforted her for a while. 'At least there is no fever, and the associated symptoms could disappear in due course,' the doctors pacified her parents. But it was nearly five days since Jiya had eaten well. She had been on liquids, intravenous drips and the best supportive medications. Yet, she was visibly getting worse. The cough made it difficult for her to sleep at night, and vomiting in the morning exhausted her.

Vomiting is a complex process that involves brain-to-muscle coordination. The causes of acute (sudden onset) vomiting in a child were many, and could only be identified with ease if doctors were highly focused. The crux was to ask the right questions. Many factors were necessary to assess causes for acute vomiting in children, such as age at presentation, the type of vomiting, and associated symptoms and signs. The doctors went through everything possible in the clinical history and finally decided that it was either pneumonia (because of the severe cough) or a gastrointestinal infection that was haunting little Jiya. But chest X-ray reports and abdominal scans came back normal. The blood counts were well within the normal range for Jiya's age, and the many markers of infection that were sent to confirm viral or bacterial causes also came back negative. But there was something extraordinary.

The liver tests.

The liver enzymes alanine aminotransferase (ALT or SGPT) and aspartate aminotransferase (AST or SGOT) were in the thousands. This was concerning. Was this all part of an evolving infectious hepatitis? The clinical presentation did fit, but the cough was strange. However, since every patient did not walk out of textbooks and the reality of clinical medical practice was very different from the world of medical books, the doctors sent a special panel to assess the presence of various viral infections to understand the cause of severe hepatitis in Jiya. These tests included blood markers for viral hepatitis A, B, C, D and E. To their surprise, all of it came back negative. The doctors were stuck between the devil and a shark-infested sea. In a fix, they thought deeply about the sudden causes of acute hepatitis presenting in a child with features of chest and abdominal infections, but with all workup for infections coming back negative, they were flummoxed.

Moreover, something sinister was happening to Jiya that no one was prepared for. Her blood glucose levels dropped like crazy, threatening her little life. She still was not eating well, and had been on intravenous drips and liquids for a while now. Her symptoms could have been due to a lack of nutrition, the doctors thought. So they increased her intravenous nutrients and oral intake as much as she could tolerate. Hypoglycaemia, or dangerously low glucose levels in a little child, is no silly matter, and the doctors knew this. The worried physicians searched for causes of severe recurrent hypoglycaemia in a child, and entered the enormously difficult-to-traverse, mind-numbingly complex realm of liver diseases in children that can present with low glucose, hepatitis and even rapid progression to death—a group of disorders known as inherited metabolic diseases of the liver.

Since Jiya was already six years old, a lot of the metabolic diseases of the liver were quickly ruled out. The presentation was too late, and her blood reports did not show the features characteristic of those disorders, such as acidosis or the elevation of levels of acid in the blood. Tests for ketones—substances produced in the liver when fat cells break down in the blood, associated with a life-threatening condition called ketoacidosis—were also negative. Other clinical features of genetic disorders were absent in Jiya. But there was still the possibility of a genetic condition called Wilson's disease (which we saw in the prologue as a possible culprit for symptoms we witnessed in another little girl, Saikrishna)—fatal when overlooked, curable when diagnosed—in which a genetic defect resulted in the accumulation of copper in the liver and brain, and children presented with liver failure that rapidly progressed to death. But then again, in Jiya's case, the screening and diagnostic tests for Wilson's disease came back negative. The doctors now had only one more disease to investigate, as Jiya's liver enzymes (ALT and AST) kept climbing and went beyond the 6,000s with the child getting even more lethargic. The only disease that needed urgent review and evaluation was a condition called autoimmune hepatitis.

When the immune system goes haywire and starts attacking the host after a trigger, or in the presence of a genetic risk, the liver is a common organ involved in such an attack. Jiya's mother's sister suffered from autoimmune liver disease, and hence, the strong family history tied Jiya's current condition to autoimmune hepatitis. But then again, the doctors were stumped. And exhausted. The screening tests and diagnostic algorithm for autoimmune hepatitis came back negative, and all the blood markers for autoantibodies, cardinal features of autoimmune hepatitis, were also negative. The limiting threshold for investigating Jiya had been reached, and the physicians caring for her did not know what had to be done next. To add to their worries, a fresh set of liver tests revealed that Jiya's AST and ALT had now crossed 8,000 U/L.

When there was no hope in sight as far as a clinching diagnosis, the doctors called it a day. They continued their best supportive care, hoping that whatever was hurting Jiya would go away in due course if the natural history of the disease was benign. But it was not so. The doctors, after much discussion, and after stabilizing Jiya on better medications for her vomiting and dehydration, provided clearance for travel by plane so that her parents, under their own responsibility and risk, could get her to a place where they hoped to find sanctuary.

Kerala.

Their home.

Being home often feels like a final comfort, a place to embrace death even when everything else was lost. In my practice, I've witnessed the bittersweet moment when patients are told they're dying, and families are presented with the option of end-of-life care.

A common question always surfaces in that dark space:

'Can we take him home?'

'Can I go home?'

'Doctor, will you discharge me so I can be home?'

At first, I wondered what home could truly offer the dying. But over time, I began to understand. It wasn't just a place—it was a final stand, a last bargain with death. 'You can take me,' I imagined them saying, 'but only on my terms and from my choice of place.' A quiet defiance, a small victory in an inevitable loss.

So I gave them that freedom. To die not in sterile halls, but in familiar surroundings, among the people and memories that shaped them. Even as their body failed, their soul found dignity and solitude in a place that held love. I always offered that choice—because to die at home was brutal, but beautiful.

If it were me, I'd want the same. Not hooked to machines in an ICU, surrounded by strangers in scrubs, but in my own bed, in my own space—knowing the end was mine to own. Who wouldn't want that?

And here was Jiya, back home and within my sanctuary, lethargic in front of me, in the cuddling fold and hold of her mother—waiting to be salvaged from something that was hurting her liver that no one could figure out. I was flustered out of my wits. Panicked inside, I kept calm on the outside.

Would I be sending Jiya to embrace the snuggle of the bittersweet, brooding night in her home, or would I be going back to mine, content that she walked back home?

Purgatorio

The doctors, in their referral summary, had mentioned that Jiya was going into ALF. Acute liver failure in children is a devastating condition that kills. If the cause remained unidentified, the chances of death or requiring a liver transplant were very high. Where would Jiya end up? Acute liver failure occurs when there is jaundice due to liver damage and abnormal thinning of the blood due to liver failure, along with another clinical complication called hepatic encephalopathy.

However, in children, especially in younger ones, early brain failure can be challenging to detect. Therefore, an accepted definition includes severe blood thinning along with jaundice, even in the absence of brain failure. Jiya's tests were bizarre. Her liver tests were through the roof, but there was no jaundice at all. Even clinically, her eyes and urine did not turn a deep yellow. The bilirubin levels were perfectly normal. So we looked at causes for very high liver enzymes in children and saw that Jiya was negative for all of them—viral hepatitis, paracetamol poisoning, shock liver (happens with circulation collapse and shallow blood pressure due to infections or bleeding) and autoimmune hepatitis.

But there was something else. Another liver test parameter, the enzyme called alkaline phosphatase, was also high; the doctors were worried about that too. Since she was a growing child, the source of high alkaline phosphatase was the bone, not the liver, which was confirmed by the presence of normal levels of another test called gamma-glutamyl transferase (or GGT). High alkaline phosphatase due to an origin from liver damage would be associated with high levels of GGT too. Again, we saw that the bilirubin levels were normal. Even though the blood tests for autoimmune liver disease were negative, autoimmune hepatitis was still a possibility considering the condition called 'seronegative autoimmune hepatitis', in which the blood tests were non-contributory.

The liver biopsy would show the classic features of autoimmune liver damage, and it was mandatory to diagnose it.

We discussed the need to biopsy the liver of this young girl with her parents. Without thinking twice, they gave us permission to biopsy little Jiya's liver, as they were tired of being unable to identify the cause of their loving daughter's disease, and her twin sister was impatiently waiting for her at home. They had nowhere else to go, and this was the place. This was their only, and last, sanctuary—a place where unconventional methods and out-of-the-box thinking would help them get to the bottom of it. Since Jiya had a high risk of bleeding due to underlying blood thinning brought on by the liver failure, we performed a transjugular liver biopsy.

Since the workup for severe hepatitis also included looking at rare infections—such as the Epstein–Barr virus, cytomegalovirus, herpes simplex and others—we sent a particular test called a polymerase chain reaction multiplex, which would help us detect multiple viruses from a single sample. Meanwhile, we held on to the hope that Jiya's diagnosis was seronegative autoimmune hepatitis, which could easily be managed with steroid therapy, and she could be sent home sooner rather than later.

At our request, the pathology department started processing Jiya's liver tissue with haste while we kept her on the best supportive treatment. We also added injectable N-acetylcysteine to her cocktail of medicines, since recent studies had showed that this supplement product helped improve survival in patients with severe acute liver injury, even in cases other than paracetamol poisoning. Jiya seemed to improve in twenty-four hours, with her vomiting ceasing and her glucose levels stabilizing.

Then, the next day, I got a call from the pathologist who wanted me to hurry to the department and see what Jiya's liver looked like under the microscope. Rushing down the stairs, ignoring the elevators, I reached the pathology central lab, where a microscope with Jiya's perfectly stained liver tissue was waiting for me.

I peeped into the microscope and saw Death looking back at me.

I looked at my pathologist, and she asked me how Jiya was doing. I told her she was doing fine. Then she said what we were both thinking, 'For how long will she be fine?'

As I kept looking into that microscope and at the condition that Jiya's liver was harbouring, I found myself descending into the innermost circle of Hell as I readied myself to battle against one of the worst liver diseases known to humankind.

A child-killer that I had only read about in my textbooks during medical training.

I was facing this demon for the first time.

Paradise

In 1963, a pathologist described twenty-one children who presented with severe vomiting, low glucose and elevated liver enzymes. These children also experienced a change in their mental status, developed altered behaviour and had varying grades of consciousness, with some of the affected progressing to coma. Of these twenty-one children, seventeen died within the first three days of hospital admission. Before the onset of this disease, each child had experienced malaise, usually associated with an upper respiratory tract infection—exactly like Jiya. By 1977, 454 such cases were reported in the US alone, and of the 373 cases of children with follow-up, 42 per cent died, while 11 per cent survived with residual brain damage. The incidence of this terrifying liver disease increased during times of seasonal viral infections and epidemics, especially the influenza-A virus infection and chicken pox outbreaks. The pathologist who identified this in 1963 was R. Douglas Reye, and the monstrosity of the disease he described came to be known as Reye's syndrome.

The syndrome most commonly only impacts children, but it affects fewer than one in a million children yearly. In the mid-1960s, after the publication of Reye's report, physicians and researchers worldwide worked to identify a cause for Reye's syndrome. As early as 1965, it was suggested that the syndrome could be caused by hypersensitivity to a group of drugs called salicylates, which included aspirin. In 1986, the US Food and Drug Administration placed a warning on all aspirin-containing products, and the warning remains on aspirin and aspirin-based formulations to this day. If you look at the back of an aspirin tablet strip, these words are notable: 'Children and teens with chicken pox or flu symptoms should not use this drug. In case of consumption, consult a doctor if behaviour changes, nausea, or vomiting occur, as these may indicate Reye's syndrome.' However, the link between aspirin and Reye's syndrome has not been conclusively proven, and this notorious link is still challenged and debated today. Although the incidence of Reye's syndrome is certainly dropping, there are reports in the literature with the majority of cases in children ending in death or liver transplantation. What I saw under the microscope was the classic Reye's syndrome–related destruction of Jiya's liver.

Reye's syndrome should be suspected in any child exhibiting a sudden onset of brain failure or encephalopathy (without known heavy metal or other toxin exposure) and persistent vomiting associated with liver dysfunction. A liver biopsy provides a definitive diagnosis, showing severe and extensive deposition of tiny fat globules packed into liver cells, along with the vast loss of liver cells within the liver tissue without any actual inflammation. This was the critical point; the pattern I saw made my heart stop transiently. My head ached, and my palms sweated. I returned to check on Jiya in her room and asked her parents how she was doing. She was sleeping, and I was worried about whether she was too sleepy, groggy or irritable. But her parents were confident she was not, and I heaved a sigh of relief.

But what had caused this?

Why did Jiya almost get to meet and greet Death while she battled one of the terrifying liver diseases known in paediatric hepatology practice?

Like clockwork, I got my answer the next day when the final reports of the virus infection panel for multiple viruses that we had sent a few days earlier popped up on my screen, while I awaited Jiya's pending results. The culprit was a rare but well-documented microbe that caused respiratory infections in children. A virus had attacked Jiya's respiratory system, given her an upper chest infection and, in the process, triggered Reye's syndrome without the use of aspirin.

A sneaky little fiend known as adenovirus.

Some children can develop adenovirus bronchiolitis (inflammation of the small airways) or pneumonia, both of which can be severe. Adenoviruses can also cause coughing fits that look almost exactly like whooping cough, or can mimic retching and vomiting in babies. Adenoviruses Types 40 and 41 can also cause gastroenteritis. A combination of conjunctivitis (inflammation of the whites of the eye) and tonsillitis (infection and inflammation of tonsil glands) is ubiquitous with adenovirus infections.

Adenovirus infections triggering Reye's syndrome are seldom reported in medical literature. Many children have died. But Jiya was holding strong. She recovered with only the best supportive care that medical science had to offer. In three days, her liver tests normalized and her appetite returned. She was bubbly and cheerfully spoke to her twin sister on video calls. There was hope in her that they would be going home. A palpable intuition that everything was going to be okay—something that only children gave off, for us to experience gleefully in silence.

Jiya had a severe but rare form of fatty liver disease called acute severe microvesicular steatosis, in which large numbers of fat droplets pack into the liver cells and damage them, leading to liver failure triggered by an event—in her case, an adenovirus infection. Fatty liver is now known as steatotic liver disease. The change in nomenclature was made to avoid stigmatizing people affected by the disease indirectly, by way of fat-shaming. Steatotic liver disease is *not* a disease but an association of a disease. Many persons, including doctors themselves, diagnose and treat fatty liver without understanding the fact that it is its cause that requires treatment, not the fatty liver per se. The most common reason for fatty liver in the world would arguably be a condition called metabolic syndrome.

Metabolic syndrome is an accumulation of several disorders that are diagnosed when a person has any three out of the following: a waist circumference of more than 40 inches in men and 35 inches in women; elevated triglycerides of 150 mg/dL or greater; reduced high-density lipoprotein cholesterol (HDL) less than 40 mg/dL in men or less than 50 mg/dL in women; elevated fasting glucose of 100 mg/dL or greater; and systolic blood pressure values of 130 mmHg or higher or diastolic values of 85 mmHg or higher. When men or women have abnormal liver enzyme ALT level in the absence of other chronic liver disease causes—with liver imaging or a liver biopsy suggestive of fat deposition in liver cells (minimum 5 per cent of total liver cells should be affected)—along with any of the above points of metabolic syndrome definition, in the absence of significant alcohol use (>50 g/day for females or >60 g/day for males), the diagnosis of metabolic-dysfunction-associated steatotic liver disease or MASLD (new terminology for NAFLD or non-alcoholic fatty liver disease) is made.

If the person had significant alcohol use, then the diagnosis would be alcohol-related liver disease. If they had features of metabolic syndrome along with 'non-problematic' alcohol use (140–350 g/week [20–50 g/day] for females or 210–420 g/week [30–60 g/day] for males), then the diagnosis would be Met-ALD—that is, both metabolic syndrome and alcohol contributing to the fatty liver deposition and subsequent liver disease. With alcohol use, more than 90 per cent of problem drinkers, who consume four to five standard drinks per day, develop fatty liver, which reverses entirely in two weeks during abstinence. Treatment of fatty liver is, in effect, the treatment for causes of fatty liver. No number of medications can improve, reduce or reverse fatty liver if causes for it remain undiagnosed, undertreated or improperly addressed. Apart from alcohol, and contrary to what people believe, fats do not make a person fat—the excess of daily calorie-dense food intake, a poor lifestyle and genetic predisposition, along with the presence of metabolic diseases do.

Alessandro dal Borro was a Tuscan nobleman and general who became the Holy Roman Empire Field Marshal for his distinguished fighting in battle. He fought many battles against the Turks and was nicknamed 'the terror of the Turks'. He finally died, aged fifty-six, due to fatal wounds received in battle against pirates. But there was something else the Tuscan General was known for. His obesity. At the time, obesity was considered a status symbol, and his portrait (*Portrait of a Gentleman,* c. 1645; an oil-on-canvas painting by French baroque artist Charles Mellin) proved the first vivid description of morbid obesity.

The first medically described documentation of fatty liver was in the year 1836 by Dr Thomas Addison, in persons with alcohol use who developed tuberculosis. In 1849, the pathologist Carl von Rokitansky described fatty liver in children who were overfed. In 1860, Friedrich von Frerichs found that not only fatty food but also excessive amounts of any food (particularly carbohydrates) resulted in fatty liver, which was more prevalent in females than males. Heribert Thaler, in 1962, first described that fatty liver can lead to progressive scarring of the liver, resulting in cirrhosis. Since then, several reports in the 1950s through the 1970s, by way of liver biopsies, documented the occurrence of fatty liver disease in obese and diabetic individuals.

It was Jurgen Ludwig, in 1980, who first described the severe form of the fatty liver called non-alcoholic steatohepatitis or NASH (now called MASH: metabolic-dysfunction-associated steatohepatitis), which was linked to severe progression to cirrhosis and the development of liver cancer. Non-alcohol-related forms of fatty liver truly did not have recommended or approved drug treatments (except, until recently, the drug called resmetirom, approved by the US Food and Drug Administration). A large proportion of treatments that doctors provided patients in the form of long prescriptions were mostly to scratch the backs of pharmaceutical companies (potentially, the drug saroglitazar with low level of evidence, but high levels of prescription) for kickbacks, or out of sheer ignorance on the ineffectiveness of certain medications (for example, the drugs ursodeoxycholic acid, milk thistle or S-adenosyl methionine, also called SAMe) in the treatment of this condition. One of the most encountered liver diseases in routine clinical practice, fatty liver disease remains one of the most poorly treated, even in the wake of overdiagnosis. Sometimes, even the most commonly identifiable and easily diagnosed fatty liver disease can still pose a significant diagnostic challenge. Some of its causes continue to stretch the limits of my diagnostic imagination, as things may not be as simple as they seem in the practice of clinical medicine.

Jiya and her parents came and saw me in the outpatient office on the day of their discharge. They were travelling out of India and back to their place of stay in the Middle East.

'So, finally, you are going home?' I asked Jiya.

'No, sir,' her mother told me, almost cutting my words off. 'We are going back to our house. This is our home.'

The Incarnate

Fatty liver disease is generally used to describe non-alcohol-related fatty liver in the layman context. However, this is not so. Fatty liver is a condition that can mimic many diseases and can be part of various diseases that primarily or otherwise also include the liver.

In 2018, when I was in my second year of specialized practice, a thirty-year-old man was brought into my outpatient department with sudden-onset liver disease—the cause for which no other physician could identify. He was jaundiced, and his liver tests were grossly abnormal. He felt weak and his appetite was poor. The man had recently joined a gymnasium and started to work out to build muscles and tone his body; he was to get married in six months. He was not taking any supplements, vitamins or other drugs, and he did not have any other known diseases for which he was on medications.

When I met him, he was skinny and underweight. But the blood and imaging report the young man's father showed me told a different story. His ultrasound revealed a massive liver with severe fat deposition.

Why was there a severe form of fatty liver disease in a young, thin man?

I was astounded.

He was a teetotaller. After we reasonably ruled out viral infections affecting the liver, systemic bacterial and parasitic infections and inherited disease conditions of the liver—and further confirming that the tox screen was clean—there was little we could gather in the context of diagnosis for his ongoing liver disease. So we did the next best thing.

We asked the liver to speak to us directly.

Through a liver biopsy.

The biopsy reports were surprising and unexpected.

Of all the young man's liver cells, nearly 85 per cent of them were extensively packed with fat globules, both large and small, giving us a confirmatory diagnosis of severe fatty liver disease—also called steatohepatitis. As we knew that fatty liver was always an associated finding and never the primary disease, we journeyed to find its cause. Every single cause—from metabolic syndrome to diseases of the thyroid to heart (cardiovascular) disorders, tests for drugs, alcohol and genetic diseases—was non-contributory.

Desperate for answers, we revisited that part of clinical medicine that held real answers, but only when the right questions were asked—the clinical history. I went back to get a detailed history from the young man himself once again, to cover all tracks and leave no loose ends. Unsurprisingly, he denied drug supplements and alcohol use again. I told him that his liver biopsy would never lie because it was conclusive of severe fatty liver disease, and the only place where we have seen that was with alcohol consumption. I offered him a discrete blood-alcohol screening test, without informing his family. It would be our little secret. But he denied alcohol use rigorously and was stubborn about the fact that he had never consumed alcohol in his life.

I was convinced.

But patients lie.

As I was about to leave the room, he asked me, curiously, 'Do food supplements count?'

I perked up and asked him what he meant by that.

He told me that he had been on a particular food supplement, which was given to him by an alternative medicine practitioner—an Ayurveda practitioner, to be clear—to improve his weight, increase his masculinity and general well-being before his proposed wedding day. He showed me the image of the 'supplement' on his phone, and the last, lost piece of the puzzle returned to complete the picture.

Narasimha Rasayana is a traditional Ayurvedic herbal butter formulation believed to rejuvenate young men. Narasimha is a fierce avatar of the Hindu God Vishnu who incarnated as part lion and part man to destroy evil and end religious persecution. Narasimha Rasayana, considered true to its name, is believed to improve manliness like the fierce God. In Ayurvedic practice, this product is also used to initiate Snehakarma, an ancient pseudoscientific practice in which oiling (external use or internal consumption) or induced sweating of a person was performed before they were subjected to a primal therapy known as Panchakarma—which includes induction of vomiting after feeding herbal decoctions, instigation of diarrhoea by consuming herbal drugs in oily liquids or by way of rectal herbal enema; and bloodletting through crude cutting of veins or arteries, or with the use of bloodsucking leeches.

Fortunately, my young patient was only advised to take the product internally and was not subjugated to the primitive monstrosities that are promoted in the name of Ayurvedic wellness. The use of the Rasayana as part of Snehakarma is believed to reduce premature ejaculation, improve weight, increase muscle strength, promote hair and beard growth and enhance intelligence—all of which remain tall claims without any evidence. Narasimha Rasayana contains many herbs, butter and milk, making it a rich source of deleterious saturated fats.

The young man feared modern medications and supplements for weight gain. He had chemophobia—the abnormal, excessive or unreasonable fear of chemicals. And as Gordon Gribbin, in his 2013 master's dissertation at Imperial College London mentions, it is a 'shared public reaction to scientific or media reports and tropes used by alternative medicine practitioners and industry' to lead people away from realistic science-based medical care and embrace supposedly 'naturally safe', unscientific or pseudoscientific therapies.

He consumed the herbal butter for almost two months before developing the current symptoms. After this Ayurvedic supplement was withdrawn and a low-calorie diet along with standard medical care for fatty liver disease were provided, expectedly, we found that his liver tests normalized in due course, over a follow-up period of four months.

During the last follow-up, his fiancée accompanied him and invited me to their wedding. I saw that she was perfectly fine with marrying a skinny young man.

On that day, I learnt that 'fatty liver' was no longer just a fatty liver.

It was always a finding, never the cause.

I understood that, in medical practice, common sense played a great role, strengthened by an act of persistent curiosity.

Things that are meant to be found will remain hidden if we choose to stop our hunt. If we do not think to ask the right questions.

Clinical medicine is not a practice, but an art; not a job, but curiosity; and there's never a dull moment, if patients are the physician's true concern.

I also learnt something important about fatty liver that day. As Miguel de Cervantes says, 'Take away the cause, and the effect ceases.'

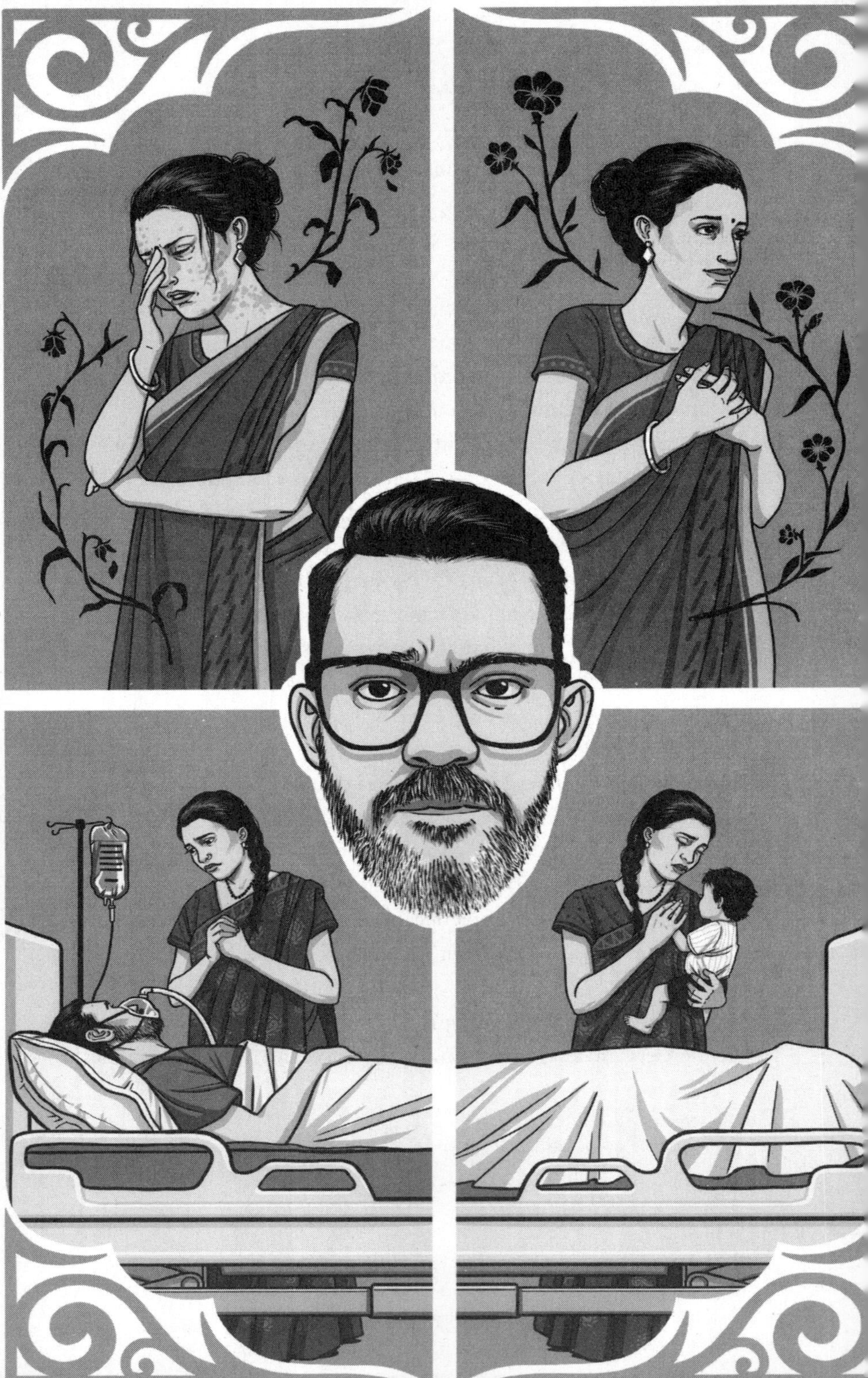

CHAPTER 8

MELANCHOLIC AND VITRIOLIC

Afflictions of the Biliary System and Bile Ducts

Melancholic

'Listen to your patient, she is telling you the diagnosis.'
—Sir William Osler

A MIDDLE-AGED WOMAN ENTERED MY OUTPATIENT DEPARTMENT room. She had been diagnosed with clinical depression six months earlier and was placed on multiple antidepressants, mood stabilizers and anti-anxiety pills long-term.

But her problems did not seem to go away.

'But I am a hepatologist,' I told her. 'I do not treat mental health disorders or depression.'

'I was told by my friends who know your work that your clinical department can diagnose me,' she answered with great hope. 'Could you please at least evaluate me?'

~

Neena was married, a mother of two children, and she and her husband both worked to keep their family comfortable. Their marriage was a loving one, and the couple were social. Except for the past twelve months, since she had started feeling the 'blues'. She did not feel like meeting people, and being home helped, but she felt lonely even when she was in the company of her family. She would step out only for an occasional dinner with family members, or a simple get-together with very close relatives. She felt tired all the time. She would go to bed early and was not interested in doing household chores or helping at home; the family had to hire a part-time maid on top of their full-time house help to assist with cleaning and other prolonged chores. Even nine hours of sleep did not restore her energy and well-being. As her tiredness worsened, her mood swings became more frequent.

When her altered mood, lack of sleep and fatigue became worse, her husband thought it was time to meet a physician and discuss her health issues. The first physician they met ran a bunch of tests and told her that it was just fatty liver and a condition called fibromyalgia, a disorder characterized by widespread musculoskeletal pain along with fatigue, and also sleep, memory and mood issues.

'Basically,' the physician said, 'you are too stressed, and there are a lot of psychological disruptions within you. A good night's sleep and daily aerobics will take care of it.'

So he prescribed her anti-anxiety pills and multivitamins. The anti-anxiety pills made her fatigue worse, and she felt groggy all day. After three weeks, the couple decided it was time to meet a psychiatrist. He spent time counselling her and then provided her with more medications, which the patient and her husband assumed would probably work better than what the physician gave her. The psychiatrist conducted extensive counselling, reviewed her baseline tests and told them the final diagnosis, and that she would get better soon.

He told her she had clinical depression and that all her symptoms were due to depression, and antidepressants would work better than anti-anxiety pills. One week into the treatment, Neena felt better than before. The antidepressants were working better than the anti-anxiety pills. But her sleep was still not restorative, and she lost large clumps of hair daily. Her mouth turned dry and her eyes felt 'gritty'.

'Probably due to the pills,' her husband reassured her.

Another visit to the psychiatrist confirmed it. Some antidepressants had adverse effects, such as dryness of mouth and eyes, and would not be a big bother in the long term. Owing to this, Neena was advised to continue the same regimen.

Weeks went by, and Neena felt like she was going to die. But she did not bother others in her family about these thoughts because she was depressed, and she felt it was all her fault—even though the source of her depression remained unidentified. She kept taking the pills the psychiatrist advised her to, and her body underwent changes that she could not explain other than by blaming the medications.

It started with the skin darkening or hyperpigmentation—first, it was her arms, then legs and finally, her neck. Over the course of a few months, the skin on her face turned dark too. Again, the pills were blamed, and everyone concurred that since she was better than before, it was prudent to wait and watch. But the real problems never went away, and Neena always felt fatigued. She was overweight, and the pills were making her gain more weight. She checked herself into a laboratory testing centre the next day for some tests and saw that her liver functions had got worse.

'The liver tests will be worse, dear,' her husband chipped in. 'You have already had fatty liver. Now there is weight gain, so it has got worse.'

According to her husband's suggestion, they both started brisk walking and jogging in the morning as part of an exercise routine aimed at shedding those extra kilos. She felt good. Not because her symptoms were getting better—they were still the same—but because now she was able to enjoy another person's company after so long. A much-needed change from the dreary home-only routine previously.

But there was another obstacle. She could not walk more than ten steps without feeling tired and, now and then, she would take long stops to catch her breath. The brisk walks were physically and mentally challenging beyond a point.

'You have to keep at it every day, and once the stamina improves, you'll touch a hundred steps in one minute, trust me,' her husband insisted.

But two weeks into the exercise and walks, she still felt breathless—exactly like how she was on the first day, maybe worse. She would get fatigued quickly in the shortest time.

Finally, the exercises stopped, and she went back to being home alone because she was too 'overweight' and 'not up to it'.

Another few months passed, and now the ordeal had become hellish. Her liver values were still high, and her skin pigmentation was worsening. But there was something new. Neena's whole body itched like crazy, mainly at night. Her already disturbed sleep was now chaotic. The more she scratched, the more the itching worsened; even when she used a sharp hair comb to itch, she was not getting any satisfaction from all that vigorous, maddening itching. When there was no hope left, the family became clueless about her and the physicians she met told her she was just becoming 'madder'.

She had come to me for a re-evaluation.

I listened, then acted.

~

I started from the beginning.

I asked her, 'Why were you depressed?'

'I was not depressed. I was tired, and I could not sleep.'

'Why could you not sleep?' I led her.

'Because something was crawling under my skin, mostly on my palms and soles, and during the nights it was terrible,' she confirmed.

While she spoke with me, I saw that she would take breaks during our conversation to take sips of water. Since our conversation started, this was the sixth time I had seen her drink water.

'Do you have diabetes?' I asked her. And she said no.

'Do you feel extremely thirsty and hungry, and do you feel like you need to pee all the time?'

She denied it.

'Then why are you drinking so much water?' I asked her.

'Because my mouth is always dry,' she told me. 'It's the medications,' she confirmed without me asking.

I asked her if the dry mouth started before or after her medications, and she was clear that it had worsened after the medications, but it had always been there months before that.

No one had asked her about it; and she thought it was because her 'body work' was such that she needed to drink much more water than others, since no person was alike.

'What about the itching?'

'It has worsened so much now since last month,' she told me.

'And the skin darkening?' I asked her. She told me it had worsened over the past three months.

I sat up because a lot of Neena's symptoms were present much before she was started on various medications, and they had slowly but steadily progressed.

Skin-darkening due to antidepressants was very rare and would only occur after many years of use, which was not her case. I asked her to show me the liver function tests that she had been doing for a while. Many physicians who saw her blamed the liver test abnormalities on a 'fatty liver'.

The liver-enzyme levels were quite intriguing. The AST, ALT and alkaline phosphatase (ALP) were all high.

'Were these always this high?' I asked her.

'No, just the ALP was initially high; the others started to rise probably in the last three months,' she added. After gaining weight, her ALT and AST started to rise, but her ALP was always above three to five times the upper limit of normal.

I had to confirm something. So I told her to get admitted.

'Let us get you off the antidepressants,' I told her as I gave her the admission note.

Alkaline phosphatase is an enzyme secreted from multiple sources in the human body. Another specific blood test called gamma-glutamyl transferase (GGT) is usually performed to identify if the ALP is of liver origin due to the small bile duct damage inside the liver. If ALP and GGT are elevated, it would be a liver-disease-related rise in ALP. If GGT is not raised, other sources for the high ALP must be looked for—including bone disorders and intestine or kidney diseases. In Neena, the GGT was highly raised. This was a clue that there was something wrong with her liver. But there was something more. The ALT and AST were also high. This meant that her liver and bile duct cells (the source of ALP within the liver) were also affected. Why were the ALT and AST raised? Was it due to the fat? Fatty liver disease can increase both enzymes, but a rise in ALP was unlikely. Were we dealing with two diseases? Or was all of this induced by the drugs she had been on for so long? Or was there just one disease that was hiding behind a lot of man-made chaos, lost in translation? On our way to find solutions, we ended up asking more questions.

One thing was clear. Neena had what we call cholestatic liver disease. It's a type of disease that affects the liver bile ducts—small or large—and causes inflammation of the bile system and stagnation to its flow within the liver, resulting in injury to liver and bile duct cells presenting as high ALP and GGT in the long term.

But what was causing it?

We went ahead with an ultrasound scan of the abdomen to look for tumours, bile duct obstruction, and gall bladder and bile duct stone disease. The scan generally returned normal, except that the liver was large and fatty. We checked for viral infections and autoimmune liver disease, both were negative in Neena's case. Meanwhile, Neena suffered from worsening dryness of the mouth and eyes—a complex symptom called 'sicca', which is classically associated with a condition called Sjogren's syndrome. This syndrome can be associated with a disease (called secondary Sjogren's) or occur in isolation without other diseases (called primary Sjogren's or Sjogren's disease). I suspected Neena had secondary Sjogren's syndrome because her liver was already affected. There was only one way to find out.

I asked her if she was willing to have a liver biopsy as the cause of all her troubles could be found through it. If we let it, the liver would speak volumes—like a little child waiting to return home from school to talk about the day's charming and not-so-charming ordeals. The biopsy was done with ease, and while we waited for the results, I slowly de-escalated Neena's antidepressants and anti-anxiety medications in liaison with our in-house psychiatrist. On the third day, my pathologist called me to give me a result that was already at the back of my mind but would change Neena's world forever.

What had started as treatments for clinical depression over a year ago ended with a diagnosis of a condition called primary biliary cholangitis, or PBC. This is a chronic, slowly progressive disease in which the bile ducts inside the liver are steadily inflamed and destroyed, leading to bile stagnation and liver cell inflammation, which progress to cirrhosis in the absence of timely diagnosis and treatment. It commonly affects women and is considered an autoimmune disease—meaning that the body's immune system mistakenly attacks the healthy cells and tissue, specifically in the liver.

Researchers believe that a combination of general and environmental factors trigger the disease, as it usually develops slowly over time. However, a marker in the blood, called the antimitochondrial antibody, gives clues about this disease, even though many patients test negative for it. This was true for Neena too, but a liver biopsy confirmed the final diagnosis. Fatigue is the most common symptom that leads to depression in many patients. In fact, in PBC, the prevalence of depressive symptoms—such as low mood, impaired thinking, memory troubles, social withdrawal and loss of interest in pleasurable activities—is very high, affecting almost 45 per cent of patients. In Neena's case, everyone focused on only treating the depression without looking for a root cause. Science-based clinical medicine was, is and always will be the only healthcare practice that can identify the root cause of a disease to direct focused treatments. The alternative medicine practitioner's trope that only practices like Ayurveda, homeopathy or naturopathy are mature enough to identify the root cause of disease is the greatest health misinformation and myth. It has misled millions of people over centuries.

Right after we had the diagnosis, we started Neena on a drug called ursodeoxycholic acid as per weight, in divided doses throughout the day, and discharged her for further follow-up and surveillance in the outpatient department.

In due course, over many months, her sleep was restored, her fatigue improved, and she was off the antidepressants and other mood-altering medications, except for an occasional sedative.

Her liver functions normalized after six months.

One day, during a follow-up visit, I struck off her occasional sedative use also from the prescription because her sleep was wonderful.

She said, 'So I was not mental after all,' and smiled.

I smiled back and told her, 'I am still not a psychiatrist.'

We both laughed it off.

With Neena's case, I realized that every patient must be heard, and that every depression was not just depression.

As Martin H. Fischer said, 'Diagnosis was not the end, but the beginning of practice.'

Vitriolic

Not every patient who enters the hospital goes back home. And not every person admitted with critical illness ends up in a mortuary. I have learnt the art of embracing the present in my clinical practice. A patient's family member would come in alone, and, in secrecy, ask me how much time the patient had left to live. I knew my limitations. I did not have the divine powers to predict someone's death. No doctors do, although some of them are quick and confidently discuss a timeline for death—unaware of the fact that there is a possibility that they themselves would not survive the day either. A predicted timeline of death is always an additional burden that families have to carry when faced with end-of-life care. When faced with that question, I always tell my patient's family that I am unsure if I will even be at my office desk tomorrow. Anything could happen to me today. If I were to live thinking about my patients' tomorrow, I would not be living at all. It would mean I was living inside their death. Today's challenges are for today, and tomorrow is a different day. We wake every day to survive the day, not the day after.

Living in the present is so important in clinical medicine because it helps me focus on challenges better. It helps me focus on my patients rather than their tomorrow.

That is how I lived in the present for Shiva's tomorrow.

~

The young wife, Leena, was teary-eyed. She looked at her husband as emergency medicine doctors masterfully put him on the ventilator. His heart was failing, breathing laboured and he was in circulatory shock. The couple did not have children.

If he passed away, she would be alone.

The medical team and I were the only ones standing between solitude and her beloved.

Three years back, at the age of thirty-five, Shiva developed pain over the right side of his abdomen without warning. This was followed by recurrent bouts of high-grade fever and severe itching all over the body. Multiple doses of paracetamol relieved the fever, but at the end of it all, he was increasingly tired; and the severe, unrelenting itching gave him sleepless nights. The first two episodes were self-limiting, lasting only three to five days. He was wary of hospitals and took symptomatic care at home. However, the third episode of fever, and the severe abdominal pain episode that occurred a few months later, shook him to the core. Afflicted with frequent rigours and chills, Shiva had become disoriented. Seeing his eyes turn yellow, Leena took him to a nearby clinic, where they ran tests and told him he had hepatitis and required higher-centre care. The itching worsened, and full-blown insomnia had set in. Shiva was miserable. At a new hospital, the doctors looked at his bloodwork and performed a liver-specific ultrasound scan. This was precisely something classically described and out of the books, and the doctors could quickly identify the cluster of symptoms.

In the late nineteenth century, the French physician Dr Jean-Martin Charcot described a condition in certain patients called 'liver fever' or hepatic fever. In 1877, the good doctor described three symptoms—including intermittent fever accompanied by chills, right upper abdominal pain and jaundice—calling it the Charcot's triad, which occurred in patients with infection in the liver. This infection was classically related to the bile ducts and was called cholangitis. In certain patients, when they got sicker, along with these three symptoms and signs, they developed shock—a condition associated with low blood pressure due to the infection spilling into the blood. Notably, along with this, there was the presence of another symptom: altered behaviour or brain dysfunction. Doctors B.M. Reynolds and Everett L. Dargan rechristened Charcot's triad to Reynold's pentad, when bile duct obstruction and infection were also found to be associated with systemic shock and brain failure—an emergency condition requiring immediate surgery at the time.

Young male. Recurrent fever. Severe itching. Painful abdomen. Jaundice.

Shiva fit the diagnosis like a perfectly placed last piece of the puzzle.

When there was itching along with jaundice, it was called cholestatic jaundice. This meant that the jaundice was, in all probability, due to block(s) within the ducts that carry bile (within the liver or outside of it). The bile duct block inside the liver was called intrahepatic cholestasis and that outside the liver extrahepatic cholestasis. There were ways to clinically know the site of the block within the affected bile ducts. Confusingly, Shiva had features of both. The next step was identifying the cause of bile duct block or injury. The liver tests showed that Shiva had raised total bilirubin, increased fraction of direct bilirubin (meaning it was liver-related) and increased liver enzymes, including ALP and GGT. This pattern, in which ALP and GGT levels increase along with jaundice, is typical of tests where the disease is considered cholestatic or related to bile-duct-cell-related liver injury.

There are many causes of bile duct damage *inside* the liver, leading to cholestatic jaundice. The common ones include infections; alcohol and the use of certain prescription drugs, such as anabolic steroids; antibiotics, such as amoxycillin-clavulanate and azithromycin; and even many supposedly innocuous over-the-counter herbal supplements. The causes for cholestatic jaundice that occurred due to bile duct cell damage or a bile duct block *outside* the liver mainly included the presence of stones and various types of cancers affecting the liver and bile ducts, as well as diseases of the pancreas leading to shrinkage of bile ducts or tumours of the pancreas causing a block of bile ducts.

In Shiva's case, the ultrasound scan showed that the bile ducts were shrunken, swollen and dilated at specific places inside *and* outside the liver. Along with clinical signs and blood investigation findings, in the absence of stones, tumours or cancers, and in the presence of bile duct changes both inside and outside the liver in a young man, only one diagnosis came to the treating doctor's mind: primary sclerosing cholangitis.

Primary sclerosing cholangitis, or PSC, is a terrible disease affecting young men in which bile ducts undergo inflammation, damage and shrinkage, leading to bile getting held up inside the liver—causing liver inflammation, progressive damage and cirrhosis in the long term. There are many causes for this strangely difficult-to-treat disease: from genetics to immune disorder to environmental factors. A bit of everything culminating and taking the shape of the disease later in life. To confirm this diagnosis, doctors perform a special kind of imaging called MRCP or magnetic resonance cholangiopancreatography. This helps identify narrowing, blockades and stones inside the bile system.

In Shiva's case, MRCP showed severe stricture formation—meaning the narrowing, beading and dilatation of the bile ducts, both inside and outside the liver—which was highly suggestive of PSC. It was time for the doctors to initiate Shiva's treatment for PSC. But the unfortunate part of this diagnosis was that PSC was a progressive disease without a cure. The only treatment was that one had to control symptoms, slow disease progression and halt life-threatening complications—such as recurrent infections due to bile blocks, bile duct cancers, stone formation, cirrhosis development and liver failure. This was performed through a strategic medical approach: risk assessment, disease staging, supportive treatment and surveillance. And so, they started working with Shiva as per the book rules.

Since there were no approved treatments for PSC, the commonly used drug was ursodeoxycholic acid (UDCA) at 8–10 mg/kg/day in divided doses. Combination therapies with steroids and antibiotics, while showing some benefit in specific disease-related complication control, are not comprehensively helpful in reversing the liver damage or halting disease progression. The biggest hurdle in patients with PSC is recurrent infections. When large bile ducts are narrowed and blocked, a procedure known as endoscopic retrograde cholangiopancreatography, or ERCP, can be easily performed by pushing a scope through the mouth and guiding a wire inside the bile duct, then placing a stent inside the narrowed bile duct to restore the flow of bile. But in Shiva's case, such large blocks in the bile ducts did not exist, and obstruction was predominantly within the liver in the smaller ducts—and repeated infections occurred inside the liver, not in the bile ducts outside it. The current infection was so severe that Shiva presented with Reynold's pentad at the initial hospital. The doctors were unable to improve his condition, and as the clinical status worsened, he was referred to us for advanced care.

~

We looked at Shiva on the ventilator. A diagnosis of PSC was accurate. There were no doubts about it. But the clinical complication that Shiva was going through, right in front of our eyes, was highly challenging. ICU medicine is nothing but evidentiary, tested knowledge, overwhelmingly and systematically applied in quick succession, to salvage the sick in good faith. Since Shiva did not have significant obstructions within the bile duct system, interventions were not feasible, and the antibiotics initiated at the first hospital were upgraded at ours. However, repeated infections (recurrent cholangitis) were one of the worst complications associated with PSC. This essentially meant that death could come early.

With repeated infections and repeated antibiotic use, more and more resistant bacteria form, and patients die of severe multi-drug-resistant infections not responding to high-end antibiotics, as that eventually leads to multiple organ failure. Shiva had already had two severe infections in the past, and the third one had landed him on the ventilator inside an ICU in septic shock—a forerunner of multiple organ failure. There was very little from a medical standpoint that one could do.

Except for one impressive life-saving measure.

A liver transplant.

In PSC, repeated infections, among other symptoms, were an indication for a curative liver transplant. But there was a challenge. Shiva and Leena only had each other. They did not have any children. There were no potential liver donors among other family members, and the ones who came forward did not match. Leena's blood group was incompatible anyway. The whole decision now came down to supporting Shiva's clinical condition as best as we could.

In the ICU, the specialists threw everything at the bugs that were killing Shiva. They were in his blood. They were teeming inside him and damaging organs as they traversed his systems. Multiple antibiotics, the best in the armamentarium, were used. Finally, Shiva's organ functions started to improve after almost seventy-two hours of the ordeal. But Shiva was far from being out of the woods. He had to be liberated from the ventilator. That would be the safe zone.

Even though things were looking up, I couldn't help but let my mind go to the dark side. How does one cope with an unexpected death? How does one feel when a beloved family member is lost without warning? What if there was no time to prepare for grief? All these thoughts went through my head. One thing was sure—I had to prepare Leena for Shiva's death very shortly. But I did not know how. But before that, I had to prepare myself to lose my patient without warning. All that effort. All that pain. All those hardships. The lost sleep and appetite. The lost hours with family thinking about the ICU.

If Shiva died inside the ICU, Leena would be all alone.

Grief is never-ending. No one gets over it. As time passes, we all bury it deep inside by creating layers of new memories over it. But each new layer is so fragile that the vital core of grief can shine through anytime when an overwhelming trigger wakes up long-buried memories. As the saying goes, 'Grief is not a sign of weakness, nor a lack of faith, but is the price of love.'

But contrary to what we expected, as the days passed, Shiva started getting better, slowly but steadily. His infection was getting controlled. His ventilator requirements came down, and he began to wake up. In a matter of eight days, he was off the ventilator and inside the wards, where he saw Leena after what felt like an eternity. They were close. So close that time stood still when they were together. Because they had only each other.

Three days before Shiva's discharge, I spoke to the loving couple regarding what the future held. Shiva was not ready for it, and he broke down after hearing about the limited time he had left to spend with his loving wife. Leena was strong because she held powerful feelings of hope, and thought that he was going to be okay. Infections would come and go, and things would be the same. There had to be something that could help them be together. Additional experimental drugs were not helpful because they would only add to the financial burden of the couple.

What was left?

We also started looking at new targets in PSC to improve patient survival.

Then I came across something recently identified as an essential factor affecting PSC's natural history and progression: intestinal bacteria.

From 2015 to 2017, five groups of doctors and clinical scientists identified that intestinal bacteria in PSC patients were different in a way that was quite harmful to the host. However, none had attempted to modulate the harmful bacteria to become the good ones, to study what would happen to said patients. There was ample evidence that in severe significant bowel infections, alcohol-associated hepatitis and inflammatory bowel disease, changing the harmful bacteria in the intestine through a healthy donor stool transplant (also called FMT, as you may recall) would help patients live longer than expected. We were already performing stool transplants to salvage patients with severe alcohol-related liver disease on a case-by-case basis in our treating unit. This was also possible in PSC patients, but none had attempted it.

Before discharge, I spoke to Shiva and Leena and told them about this new but experimental treatment option called healthy donor stool transplant. We did not have any protocol—so we made an arbitrary one for Shiva. We would give him a fresh stool transplant from a healthy donor—once every week for four weeks through an endoscopy procedure. The processed stool suspension would be infused into the upper part of his small intestine (duodenum) through an endoscope. Shiva and Leena looked at me for a while, astonished at this strangely nauseating therapy, and then nodded their heads. Shiva would be discharged, they would find a stool donor and we would start within a week.

After a week, Shiva came with his niece. She was planned to be the healthy donor, and we performed clearance tests to assess her fitness. She got through all the test hoops and was finally cleared.

We began the process.

We pushed 200 ml of freshly processed stool suspension through an endoscope into a sedated Shiva once weekly for four weeks. We checked his liver tests and the emergence of new infections due to PSC. Weeks passed, and then months.

To our great astonishment, it paid off. Through a high-end analytical method called metagenomics, we found that the donor stool bacteria overwhelmed the bad bacteria inside Shiva's intestines. In due course, they took over, annihilating the bad bacterial groups, thereby reducing Shiva's risk of severe repeated infections and related complications. Months became a year. Shiva remained infection-free and without fever as his liver tests remained stable.

This was something new. We had done it—the first stool transplant for PSC was in a patient who earlier needed a curative liver transplant and was dying due to repeated infections. We published Shiva's report as the first on stool transplantation to control severe infections in PSC patients shortly after that, in a peer-reviewed medical science journal. After our report was published, a group of clinical scientists in the US performed stool transplants for PSC in more patients and found that it was safe and improved liver tests. But the best news was yet to come.

During one of the follow-up visits, Shiva came to my outpatient department with his cousin. Leena was missing during the review for the first time. He gladly told me that Leena was pregnant with their first child, and how they were excited. It was happiness all around.

They got me sweets. And I wished them the best.

But life is unpredictable.

Every peak has a valley.

It was time for all of us to slide down the peak and enter the valley, without warning.

~

At the end of one year, Shiva started developing fever and jaundice again. The effects of the stool transplant started to wear off. Leena wanted to try another session of the stool transplant, but Shiva wanted a permanent solution. With the child coming, they could spare very little to upgrade his treatment. With the help of many good-hearted people around them, Leena and Shiva raised money for us to work him up and get the necessary clearances to list him in the deceased donor liver transplant programme. Shiva survived longer than was expected from him—with repeated infections and hospitalizations over many months, but none as severe as the one that nearly put him in the sights of Death a year earlier. All because of an experimental therapy he was willing to undergo—bound by evidence in medicine, held up by a group of physicians who were willing to take the risk and think out of the box for their patients.

But then an episode of severe cholangitis entered like a thief in the night into our beautifully framed picture, almost two years after Shiva underwent an experimental but life-changing stool transplant. Shortly after that, Shiva died under my watch, not responding to antibiotics as new resistant microbes—this time led by extremely damaging fungi, which feasted on his organs—took him away in the same ICU where my treating team had previously fought to save his life.

Leena knew we had done everything for him.

She was with him, holding his hands when he passed away.

She was with him as he withered into the night.

They did say their goodbyes.

We gave them that chance.

The art and practice of medicine did.

This time, she was not alone. Her little daughter, whom they named Shivani, waited for her mother outside our ICU while she bittersweetly and lovingly said goodnight and a final goodbye to Shiva.

As Paulo Coelho said, 'If you are brave enough to say goodbye, life will reward you with a new hello.'

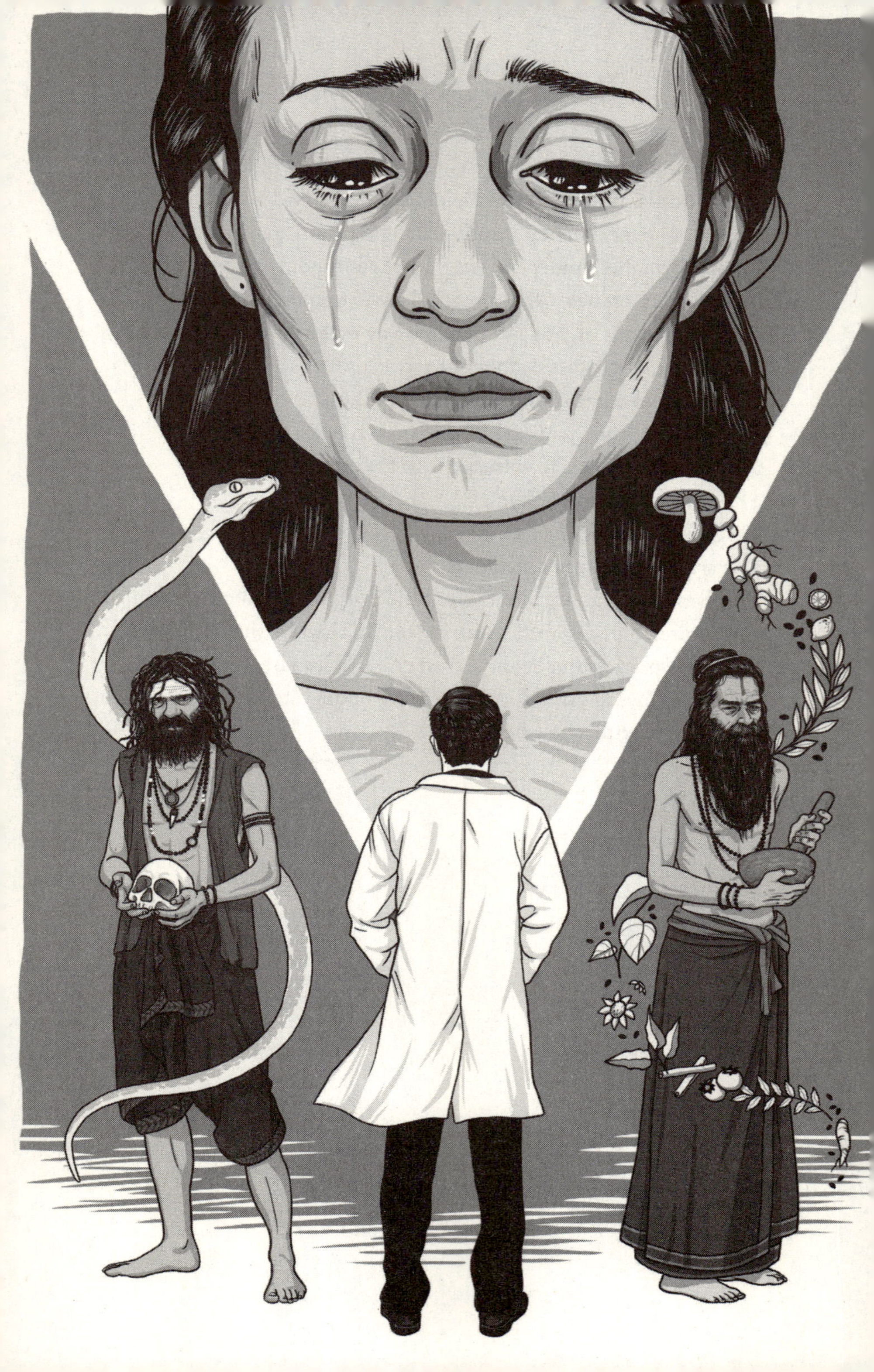

CHAPTER 9

Natural Ways to Die Unnaturally

Drugs, Toxins and Herbal- and Dietary-Supplement-Induced Liver Injury

The Longest Journey

'You know what they call alternative medicine that's been proved to work? Medicine.'
—TIM MINCHIN

'THERE IS A PLACE, BUT IT IS A LONG JOURNEY,' SAID HIS friend. 'If there is any hope for your jaundiced father, this place holds it.'

'Where is it?' the young man enquired.

'It is in Kerala. A place called Kochi.'

A son.

A dying father.

A terrifying battle.

A terrible liver disease.

From Telangana to Kerala.

A few months ago, Deepak, a middle-aged man, lost his appetite one fine day. As days progressed, he felt lethargic and every small task became a chore. Hailing from a small town in Telangana, with a small family, he was taken to a local doctor. Deepak's homemaker wife looked after their family with love and motherly care. He was the sole breadwinner, and the couple shared two children. His daughter had only recently started medical school in the private sector and had to pay hefty fees, and his son was about to join an engineering college.

Deepak had toiled hard for decades to save money so his children could get an education. Their success was his dream. He had done what he thought was impossible through honest, hard work. He saved enough to send his daughter to medical school and his son to an engineering college. The whole family, especially Deepak, lived contentedly with the simplest things. When he showed signs of illness, everyone was worried. He had never got seriously sick before, and had managed every minor illness on his own because he did not want to spend money unnecessarily at the hospital. He saved every bit for his children's future.

The severe lethargy was followed by progressive leg swelling and weight gain. Once a thin man, Deepak now looked bloated. His abdominal girth increased, and his legs swelled like balloons—so much that the skin had become taut, thick and folded like an elephant's. This made it difficult for him to walk. Basic tests at a nearby hospital did not show kidney failure, but then, progressively, his abdomen started to swell too and then ballooned even more.

This worried the family, especially his son, Vimal. Within a few weeks, he was to join the engineering college. Vimal took his father to a doctor, who looked at him carefully and ordered tests, including an abdomen scan, which revealed something they were not expecting. Fluid inside the abdomen and an abnormal liver test, with jaundice.

'Does your father drink?' the doctor asked Vimal casually. Vimal told him that his father did not. The last time he had had a standard drink was at a family function eight months earlier.

'We will run some tests,' the elderly doctor told Vimal. 'We have to find the cause for his jaundice.'

Deepak was admitted. A multitude of tests later, the doctors were flustered and confused. Everything—from viral infections, alcohol, other prescription medicines (such as the overconsumption of paracetamol), painkillers, systemic infections (such as malaria) and autoimmune liver disease—every test they did to get to the bottom of the jaundice had come back negative.

Worse, the jaundice was progressing.

As the jaundice progressed, so did the worsening of symptoms. Deepak became emaciated. His muscles were wasted and the swelling in his abdomen increased, while his oedematous legs got thicker. Water pills took care of the swelling, but the jaundice was relentless.

'We have nothing more to offer here,' the doctor told Vimal.

He nodded solemnly.

'It would be better if you can take him to a specialized liver centre—where they can figure out what is hurting his liver, causing this liver failure and if required, an early liver transplantation,' the physician assured Vimal.

But there was no time for that.

No luxury for something like that.

Vimal had to join his college. It would mean he could lose a whole year and probably the meritorious hard-earned seat. He had to deposit the fees and transfer funds. But now, all that money was being diverted towards caring for his loving father.

Deepak was suffering from a disease that was slowly eating up their money, and this was without a diagnosis. Without wasting any more time or thought, Vimal took Deepak to one of the biggest liver centres in the country—in Chennai, in south India itself. The liver specialists at Chennai re-evaluated Deepak, who was now visibly deeply jaundiced and fatigued. His bilirubin was 35 mg/dl (normal was less than 1). A review of all investigations and reassessment for rare causes of acute liver injury—including strange and rare infections that caused hepatitis—were negative. When the initial exhaustive testing becomes non-contributory in acute liver disease, the only way to understand what is happening inside the liver is to directly ask the liver itself.

A liver biopsy would provide solutions and, at times, more questions.

So Deepak underwent a liver biopsy.

The results were astonishing.

Everybody, from pathologists and junior doctors to senior consultants, developed palpable anxiety when they noticed the findings under the microscope.

A terrifying liver disease with almost 100 per cent fatality. It is so rare that no drugs work on it.

Way back in 1920, when some groups of people in South Africa developed severe liver disease and died, the mysterious cause was found to be the flavoured tea they were consuming. A specific flowering plant, called senecio, belonging to the daisy family, was used in its preparation.

What this plant and its chemicals, called pyrrolizidine alkaloids, did to the liver was terrifying. These natural compounds damage and destroy the small veins inside the liver—leading to extensive obstruction to blood flow in the large organ—resulting in massive swelling, loss of liver cells and a failure of regeneration. The subsequent liver disease that develops is called hepatic veno-occlusive disease or VOD.

There are many causes for VOD. It can be the complication of high-dose chemotherapy given before a bone-marrow transplantation, and has been described as part of a rare hereditary disease called hepatic VOD with immunodeficiency (which results from mutations in the gene coding for the human protein called SP110). Features of hepatic VOD include weight gain, painful enlargement of the liver, fluid in the abdomen and jaundice. The diagnosis is based on the recognition of the clinical manifestations and their association with a potential cause (such as exposure to pyrrolizidine alkaloids), together with the exclusion of other causes of liver disease. Liver biopsy is often indicated to confirm the diagnosis of VOD—which is now called SOS, or sinusoidal obstruction syndrome.

The doctors turned to Deepak and Vimal and, with much difficulty, told them about the morbid diagnosis.

There was no other way.

Deepak had to undergo a liver transplantation to survive. In severe cases, the prognosis was abysmal, with a high mortality rate (up to 90 per cent) due to multiple organ failure. His disease was severe, and it was only a matter of time before he landed in the ICU with progressive liver failure and multiple organ failure.

The family had no money.

Deepak needed continued admission and medical care.

Vimal made the dire decision to drop a year of college.

He used that educational fund to continue his father's treatment. Desperate times.

They left Chennai and returned home to the best supportive care, to consider their current circumstances. There was one drug available for SOS, and it was called defibrotide—but it was costly, and a cure with this drug was not guaranteed in severe cases. Transplantation was expensive but curative and the best guarantee they had. His father was going to die without a liver transplant. This was almost a surety. As the jaundice increased, a friend guided a desperate Vimal.

'There is a place,' the friend told Vimal, 'but it is a long journey. If there is any hope for your father, this place holds it.'

'Where is it?' Vimal enquired.

'The Liver Institute, in Kochi.'

~

When I met Vimal, his father's total bilirubin level (representative of clinical jaundice) was 40 mg/dl. Such high jaundice could shut down the kidneys from a complication called bile cast nephropathy, in which the bilirubin deposited inside the kidney damages the organ tissue and obstructs urine formation, flow and function. I looked at Deepak's reports and saw that his clinical situation was worse than we had thought. It was indeed SOS, and it was going to kill him. I talked to them about the seriousness of the matter. A liver transplant was imperative. But they had no money for a transplant, and the treatments were gnawing into Vimal's college fund.

Vimal's parents were a love match. Married from different castes within the same religion, they had no support from other immediate family members. No one would come to their aid. And without the money, there could not be a transplant. But medical science is not only about diagnosing and treating. It is also about caring.

I could not imagine what Vimal would have been going through—helpless, watching every day as a parent withered away right in front of his eyes, with absolutely no power to stop or change what was incoming. But how did an utterly healthy man suddenly develop a monstrous liver disease? The answer lay in the two weeks before his symptom onset.

Deepak had always harboured an anxiety disorder. His heart would race and his pulse would gallop. He was not keen on consuming medications, especially anti-anxiety drugs, as he felt they were too strong and that he would get dependent on them. So, at the behest of 'friendly' advice, he met a traditional Ayurvedic healer who performed an ancient form of evaluation called 'nadi pariksha' or pulse diagnosis. This is a primitive method described in pseudoscientific Ayurvedic texts, in which the practitioner would diagnose a host of diseases without rational investigation and only based on the type and character of the pulse. For his anxiety disorder, the traditional healer gave Deepak herbal formulations as treatment. He took the herbal products for two whole weeks and, from the third week onwards, started developing severe symptoms that resulted in the need for a liver transplant at present.

Many commonly found and prescribed herbs contain pyrrolizidine alkaloids that can harm its users. Homeopathic plant-based remedies and Ayurvedic herbal formulations contain many such plant components that can trigger severe SOS in consumers. A very commonly used herb in Ayurvedic practice belongs to the Crotalaria species: sunn hemp or smooth crotalaria. Traditional healers prescribe it, and it is well known to promote severe liver injury and liver failure, with the advent of SOS in the liver.

The diagnosis of herbal liver injury is one of exclusion, and unique scoring methods are used. We ruled out every other possible competing cause for Deepak's liver injury again and, with the help of a liver biopsy, diagnosed with a conclusiveness that the liver injury was due to traditional herbals recently given for his anxiety disorder.

An ignorant act of using traditional herbal medicines unscientifically had broken a family apart—mentally, physically and financially. And there was nothing anyone could do about it. I had to accept it now. That Deepak was going to die, and the children were going to lose their father.

Deepak needed a life-saving liver transplant. Vimal, his son, was a perfectly matching donor. Money was the only obstacle. So I started a process that would maybe help them achieve what we wanted and they needed. I relentlessly spoke with the hospital management to see if the transplant could be done free of cost. Eventually, the management buckled. I was astonished. I asked and confirmed, and they told me, 'The patient's family will have to pay zero rupees.'

Sure enough, the hospital management graciously decided to provide the liver transplant procedure utterly free of cost to Deepak and his family. After all, to serve those who come for help is a hospital's primary functioning core principle, as the right to health is for all. I felt like my department was the last line of defence against this terrifying disease that stood directly in line, with its sights on Deepak and his family. We had to go the distance.

I rushed to Vimal and asked him to get transferred to our transplant surgery unit, where his fitness would be assessed in record time. To prevent kidney injury by drastically (but temporarily) reducing jaundice, we performed a procedure called plasma exchange for Deepak. Everything was done for free. There is no clinical medicine without humanism. The fitness workup was completed in three days, and Deepak and Vimal came under the knife together—one giving a part of himself to save the other. Deepak's herbal-damaged liver came out, and a part of Vimal's healthy liver went in. The whole process proceeded smoothly and as planned. Vimal recovered and thrived after surgery. His father was shifted to the room from the ICU after a brief period of rehabilitation. As he recovered, Vimal's dream of pursuing higher studies became a reality.

He was free.

Because we did not burden the family financially.

There is a place, but it is a long journey.

If there is any hope for your father, this place holds it.

A sacrifice.

A terrifying battle won.

A terrible liver disease forgotten.

From Kerala to Telangana.

Everybody Lies

A young man, Arul, was referred for spiking fevers and abnormal liver tests, which had been going on for two weeks. He had no jaundice, but his liver values were highly elevated and it did not seem like they would come down. Doctors elsewhere were baffled, and his parents were worried as hell for the young man, since he had just joined a new job with an illustrious company in Bengaluru (previously Bangalore). For three weeks, he had been on medical leave, and his career was at stake. Whatever this was, we had to get it diagnosed quickly and get it over with so that this man could retain his job.

~

All was well until three weeks ago, when Arul started to feel lethargic. Slowly but steadily, his appetite reduced, and he began to not only lose weight but also interest in his work. He felt that office calls were a pain, and all he wanted to do was sleep. A visit to a nearby general practitioner ended with some vitamin prescriptions that did not improve his condition. As he started to feel worse, he took the overnight bus to his hometown of Palakkad in Kerala and, along with his parents, visited a senior physician near their home. His parents were concerned; he was their only child. A battery of tests was sent to look for reasons for the sudden loss of appetite, including a screening for metabolic diseases. Everything except the liver tests came back non-contributory. There was only evidence for inflammation of the liver. The tests were suggestive of severe hepatitis, in which the liver enzymes were high, but there was no jaundice.

Simple, the doctors thought.

Now, it was only a matter of finding the cause of hepatitis, and there were so many categorically specific blood tests that would help them quickly identify reasons for Arul's abnormal liver functions. They ordered tests for viral infections and blood markers to identify autoimmune liver disease, bile duct disease, liver tumours and other systemic diseases that could affect the organ—including severe infections, such as malaria, leptospirosis, rat fever and dengue. Arul was started on supportive medications to improve his liver functions, and care was taken to reduce his symptoms.

But to everyone's surprise, every test they sent out came back negative. As awful as they had been already, the liver values were significantly worsening. Then there was also a challenge with the ongoing fever, which was initially low-grade but slowly progressed to high-spiking episodes late at night. It had to be an infection; the doctors were sure. It was not a typical infection, but something strange.

So further tests for rare, atypical viral infections such as those caused by cytomegalovirus, herpes, varicella zoster, parvovirus and human immunodeficiency virus were all sent out. At one point, the doctors were thoroughly distraught that they were shooting arrows into the dark—testing for everything, hoping to get a hit on something. But they got nothing apart from the still worsening liver tests and persisting fevers. Now, the elderly physician who was in charge was overwrought.

So many tests were ordered, the bills were mounting but no answers were in sight. Arul's parents were getting impatient. As the fevers were becoming more numerous and the abnormal liver tests persisted, the senior physician knew what this was, and he felt the raging heat of the moment. It was something so stressful for a treating doctor, and it was also one of the worst situations that a physician had to face in clinical medicine: a condition called fever of unknown origin, or FUO (as discussed earlier in the book). He knew this was the time for expert opinions, as the situation was getting out of his team's hands. There had to be some input from the medical specialities. And so, a confused Arul and his worried parents were transferred to us for additional evaluation.

~

A review of all the previous reports was done at our facility. The only repeat evaluation we did was a CT imaging of the abdomen and chest so as not to miss any evolving tumours or foci of infection. Unfortunately, however, these did not show anything abnormal.

We thought long and hard about it and understood that the most complex problems always had the most straightforward solutions. We were completely taken aback looking at all the exotic tests performed at the hospital earlier. There was one persistently abnormal organ system, but no one had bothered to ask about it. So we decided that we were going to forget about all the other systems and focus on the liver. It was time to go right to the source—a liver biopsy was done.

A few days passed, and then I got a call from the senior pathologist who said, 'Ask the patient for his drug history.'

I said that we had done so, multiple times. No prescription drugs, no herbal formulations, no exotic medications or implicating food and dietary supplements—everything was negative.

My senior pathologist, a brilliant woman with years of experience in getting to know the liver up close and personal, told me, 'No, ask for *drugs*. As in recreational and psychotropic drugs.'

I sat back on the chair because we had never thought about this. Arul's father was a pastor. He was very religious and ran a church congregation, and Arul was a pious young man who was supposedly the most sociable member of their whole family. He had undergone schooling and college in Kerala with top honours, and everybody loved him for his persistent streak of 'niceness'. He never got into trouble and never got others into trouble. He had only recently shifted to Bengaluru and was free. Possibly wild, too, because the pathologist told me things that no one would believe, if it was not for the liver telling us about it.

The liver biopsy had some strange features.

Minimal areas of inflammation.

Small veins damaged.

Specific loss of liver cells at Zone 3 (the liver has, functionally, three zones).

All microanatomical structures in the central part of the liver, called the portal area, were inflamed and dying.

And I remembered.

Everybody lies.

~

I waited for my outpatient work to end. When the visiting time at the hospital was closed, and Arul's bystander, a family member, had gone out to get some water, I sneaked into his room.

Surprised to see me, he asked, 'How are you, doctor?'

And I smiled and nodded to convey that I was okay.

'How are you doing?' I asked him.

He said he was getting better, but that he was worried about what had caused his condition. He was worried that even if it got better, it might come back later.

I told him that the recurrence of this disease in his liver would entirely depend on him and him only. He looked surprised.

I asked him directly, 'What drug were you on?'

He said he had not been on anything except what the doctors had prescribed.

I looked at him, poker-faced but also empathetic, because he knew his lie had been caught.

And then he started crying right in front of me.

A grown man.

He confessed to what had happened a week before he had started feeling sick.

Cocaine use can lead to a multitude of adverse effects, including the blocking of heart vessels, abnormal heart rate and rhythm, strokes and bleeding in the brain; seizures, blocks of the blood vessels in the intestine and gangrene of the gut; kidney failure; the melting of muscles, leading to a condition called rhabdomyolysis; and, finally, a rare, acute liver injury that is almost always overlooked. It customarily arises within hours to a few days after heavy use of cocaine. Initially, in overdose, the liver enzymes rise. Most cases are self-limited, the recovery is rapid and liver tests usually return to normal within one to two weeks. However, this was not happening with Arul.

And we found out why—3, 4-methylenedioxy-N-methamphetamine, or MDMA.

There was concomitant use of the commonly known recreational psychoactive drug Ecstasy or Molly. This young man had, along with his work colleagues, who were also his newfound wild-and-free friends, snorted cocaine as well as consumed Molly, during a trip to Nandi Hills. Cocaine-induced liver toxicity, which is well documented in humans and well-studied in rodents, ranges from mildly elevated liver enzymes with or without jaundice to severe liver disease associated with multiple organ failure. It is a significant but overlooked cause for something also quite rare but still possible, a 'drug-induced fever'. The liver-biopsy findings were very classical, and any trained eye, like my senior pathologist, could quickly figure out what was hurting the liver just by peeping into the microscope. The liver-injury pattern and type of damage were very different from viral hepatitis or alcohol-related hepatitis, or other medications that can cause hepatitis.

I learnt that day that FUO, along with unexplained elevated liver levels, warranted exhaustive history-taking, focused on drug history. Not just any prescription drugs or supplements but recreational drugs too. Of course, Arul improved substantially with a short course of steroids that took care of his liver inflammation and then did a whole lot of counselling. Even when he begged me to keep this a secret from his parents, I did tell them about the entire drama that led to this mystery and mayhem. I told them in a way that made them understand that it was not their or Arul's fault that got him into trouble.

We all make mistakes.

To forgive ourselves and not repeat them is what makes us humane.

But to repeat them is also what makes us human.

I called it a day, got into my car and drove home.

We had done it.

We had served.

S(n)orted out a problem.

As Sir William Osler said, 'Medicine is a science of uncertainty and an art of probability.'

The Child on the Ventilator

A six-year-old girl was rushed into the emergency room in an unresponsive state. Chubby and cute, her innocent and pretty face was mauled by the deepest jaundice. As I watched the emergency team push a tube into her windpipe to protect the child's airways, my heart raced and my palms sweated as I entered a realm of clinical medicine that I knew would stretch my limits, make me go dark, damage my mental health—one where there was everything to lose.

Nasreen, the child, was healthy and playful until six weeks earlier. It had all started with a benign cough and low-grade fever. 'Nothing serious,' the general physician who saw her first told her parents and prescribed her cough syrup and low-dose paracetamol, as required. The fever settled, but the cough did not disappear, and cough syrup prescriptions were modified. As the cough settled in due course, two weeks later the child started to lose her appetite and refused to play with other children. She always wanted to rest, and the bed became her best friend. A week later, her parents noticed that Nasreen had yellow discolouration of her eyes, and her urine was getting quite dark—a deep yellow, as if someone had mixed turmeric in it. She had become jaundiced. She was rushed to the nearby clinic, where they evaluated her for sudden-onset causes of jaundice. Viral infection-related hepatitis was negative, and other respiratory viruses—strange but rare viruses that attack the liver, such as herpes, the Epstein–Barr virus and adenovirus—were all checked for but came back negative.

Even though she improved slightly from a fatigue point of view with all the fluids going in, her jaundice deepened, while her food intake progressively worsened. The doctors then decided to place a feeding tube through her nose and into the stomach to feed her, so that she could get some energy to battle the unknown illness and to give them some time to identify what was damaging her liver. They looked for non-infection-related causes too. The markers for autoimmune liver disease in the blood were, again, negative. As her jaundice worsened, the child started to behave weirdly and, in due course, became disoriented. She could not identify her parents. The doctors knew what this was, and they shuddered at the thought of it. Jaundice, followed by altered behaviour (hepatic encephalopathy) in quick succession, meant that Nasreen had gone into a terrifying disease condition called acute liver failure or ALF.

As discussed in earlier sections, ALF is a condition in which a perfectly healthy liver fails due to an acute insult, with a high death rate due to multiple organ failure in the short term. The only curative option was a liver transplantation. Without wasting time, they referred the child urgently to a higher centre in order to salvage her life. But by the time she reached us, she was already in a coma and was immediately put on the ventilator to preserve her little life.

This was now no more the clinical practice of medicine. It had become a race against time. In ALF, finding the cause is of utmost importance. In ALF, time is life.

So, without delay, a liver biopsy was performed, asking the liver to speak to us directly about what was hurting it. Meanwhile, other culprits were investigated, and the test for every infectious cause we rechecked came back negative. Repeat imaging, a workup for bacterial and other rare but possible liver infections, the test for the genetic condition called Wilson's disease (in which copper overload in the liver results in liver failure in children), and screening for rare metabolic diseases that affected the liver in small children were all negative. We were unable to find clues that helped us to hold on to hope, and we were distraught. Then, finally, the liver-biopsy results came.

The pathologist told me, 'Doc, this looks like autoimmune damage to the liver, but it's not the classic autoimmune hepatitis that I expected it to be. I am seeing so many other changes in the liver that I do not understand. It's a mixed bag, so many things going on.'

She paused and then asked, 'Was she on any drugs? Anything we missed?' This led me to re-examine the clinical history. We went back to the drugs little Nasreen was previously on. There was salbutamol syrup, levocetirizine, the occasional paracetamol and a medicine called ambroxol for cough—but none were liver-toxic!

I told my pathologist with confidence, 'Drugs and supplement use were still non-contributory to her current state.'

But she was adamant that it had to be a drug-induced liver injury because the pattern of liver injury was so mixed up on the biopsy that only drugs attacking the liver would present that way.

Another session with Nasreen's mother ensued. This time, we did not specify drugs or supplements but asked her if the girl was given anything other than what the physicians prescribed for cough. A long and hard thought later, she sheepishly confirmed something that woke up our deepest fears.

Nasreen had been given a homemade herbal juice to ease her persistent cough after syrups had failed to help. At the advice of a local Ayurvedic practitioner, her mother gave her about 40 ml per day for three weeks. The herb used was *Tinospora cordifolia*, known as giloy or heart-leaved moonseed—a plant often considered 'safe' simply because it is natural and has been used over centuries in ancient medicine. But when we investigated, it opened a Pandora's box.

We had previously seen giloy trigger severe liver damage in adults, often resembling autoimmune hepatitis, but this was the first time we encountered such a severe case in a child. Far from being a 'heavenly elixir', as named in Hindu mythology, giloy was killing Nasreen. Scientific studies have shown that giloy can activate the immune system in a way that causes it to attack the liver, leading to herb-induced autoimmune hepatitis—a mix of both herbal liver-injury and classic autoimmune damage. In Nasreen's case, the diagnosis was clear. Giloy had triggered the hepatitis that led to her acute liver failure.

India has seen more than a hundred such cases, some fatal, where patients with previously stable or silent autoimmune liver disease deteriorated rapidly after giloy use. Despite clear evidence and repeated warnings, the Ayurveda community and related regulatory bodies refused to acknowledge the risk. Instead, they issued misleading press releases through government channels, falsely claiming giloy was safe, even though no quality human safety studies existed.

The Press Bureau of India's fact-check division misled the public by citing rodent studies as evidence of safety. Meanwhile, the Liver Research Club India, a credible group of physicians, documented the country's most extensive giloy-related liver-injury cases. I personally wrote to the Prime Minister's Office, presenting scientific evidence and urging the Ministry of Ayush and the Ministry of Health to issue public warnings, especially for those with autoimmune conditions.

The reply did come, not from an Ayurveda expert, but from a homeopathy practitioner within the Ministry, citing ancient Ayurvedic texts to defend giloy's use. While a few responsible health journalists covered the issue, most mainstream media stayed silent, likely to protect the Ayurvedic business ecosystem and their own ad revenues.

As for Nasreen, there were moments when we thought we would lose her. Her liver wasn't healing, and she was slipping deeper into organ failure. I lay awake at night wondering if she would survive or suffer fatal brain herniation, a devastating complication of ALF. Watching my own children at home filled me with a heavy sorrow, knowing her parents sat waiting outside the ICU, clinging to hope. But I couldn't afford to collapse emotionally—I shelved my grief and focused on fighting for her life.

I wondered about Nasreen's parents. My life would be empty if my children were hurt or sick. I would become a shell of my former self. I was slowly getting inside that madness as I lost my mind in the thoughts of cute little Nasreen, reflecting her condition upon my own children. This child had to get back home, and I was the one shouldering that burden.

Liver transplantation was never a feasible option for her family. The father ran a small shop and the mother worked as a house help on the weekends. They did not have a matching donor, and liver transplantation was an emergency that they could never realize. After we found that it was giloy juice that was harming the child's liver, we did the best we could do from a medical standpoint—we unleashed the most impressive supportive care that would help Nasreen's immune system fight the disruption giloy invited into her body. We put her on high-dose immunosuppressants after getting consent from and notifying the parents that it could also become a double-edged sword. The high, but life-saving, level of immunosuppression use could invite dreadful, opportunistic infections—such as deadly multi-drug-resistant bacteria and terrifying viruses, which would make the liver failure feel like a Sunday picnic. But they had no other options left and concurred with the only plan we put forth.

Three days of high-dose injectable steroids, and on the fourth day, Nasreen woke up on the ventilator. Dazed, confused and scared, she was taken into confidence by the expert ICU team. They taught her how she needed to breathe on her own so that they could remove the ventilator support. But she had to show them she was strong and wanted to go home. That little child with a lion heart did exactly what she was told. Home was in her mind, and everything bad around her and in her ceased to exist in those moments. She was removed from the ventilator after another six days and shifted to a room in the hospital for further rehabilitation. She was then discharged after spending three weeks in the hospital and had fully recovered in a little over eight weeks.

On one of the follow-up visits, I found her smiling as she was about to leave my outpatient room, and I asked her what she found funny in my room.

She did not answer, but her mother did.

'She is happy but so shy seeing you, doctor,' the mother told me.

A little girl who had always hated and feared hospitals was happy to see me.

'She likes coming to this hospital only … likes to see your face.' She smiled. 'She feels safe around you. Protected.'

I smiled back at them as they walked out of my outpatient room.

Then I sat down and enjoyed the minute of silence that had flooded my room.

I could not hear the beeps, clicks and whirring of machines.

There was no smell of blood, sweat or fluids.

There was no sound of Death.

Only the sigh of Life.

As Irving Berlin said, 'The song is ended, but the melody lingers on.'

Jesus Saves

'The next patient is a nun, Sister Christy, referred from DM Hospital,' a member of my outpatient staff told me. 'A case of severe hepatitis without a cause.'

I sat up, excited but also terrified.

I was excited to serve the people who brought me into this world.

Terrified because they were more than competent enough to diagnose any cause of hepatitis, but could not.

A sinister feeling loomed.

The nuns at DM Hospital had ensured my mother was taken care of when she delivered me many decades before. They were pleasant, caring and comforting. The hospital was well known for its services. A direct referral meant this was not a run-of-the-mill case; something was wrong or challenging. I watched as two nuns, seated in front of me, showed me a liver test—the liver test enzymes were in the thousands, and they described a hint of jaundice.

'I was a young nun when you were born,' the elder-looking nun told me. The doctor-nun, the one who bought me into this world, the senior nun at the time, had passed away a few years ago. But they all remembered me and my family, and my presence here gave them hope. After hundreds of tests at their specialized centre, the physicians did not have a clue about what was happening to Sister Christy's liver.

The cause for her hepatitis was as enigmatic as the presence of God.

Her past clinical history was a complicated and complex maze of medical interventions and disease diagnoses, and it was challenging to get to the bottom of what was real and unreal about her current illness.

~

Many years ago, Sister Christy had started developing weakness in one leg, which progressed over months and led her to walk with incredible difficulty. She developed a clumsy gait and her behaviour slowly changed. Extensive tests were done then, and only one result stood out. Her brain had 'white-matter changes'.

The brain is broadly composed of white matter and grey matter tissues, each with unique functions. When various insults—such as genetic mutations, inflammatory causes, infections and immune disorders—affect the white matter, patients develop many problems.

The doctors got going with a battery of tests while Sister Christy was progressively deteriorating. At the end of that long-drawn process called diagnostic evaluation, they finally concluded that she had post-infection-triggered, auto-immune-related acquired white matter disease—a rare cause for white-matter inflammation and degeneration of the brain. To combat the severe illness, Sister Christy was put on powerful medications that suppressed her immune functions and helped reduce further brain damage.

Immunosuppression works like magic in autoimmune disorders, and within weeks, Sister Christy was walking again with zest. However, steroid therapy, used as one of the mainstays of immunosuppressive treatment, was not wholly recommended to be given in the long term due to various concerns of adverse effects on the body. So, the good doctors, to protect her from the side effects of steroid therapy—in the true spirit of the realistic practice of medical science, which always aims to comfort but never exploit the patient—started reducing steroids by adding a new agent that would have action like steroids, but without its known significant side effects.

Enter the drug mycophenolate mofetil, or MMF, an immunosuppressant that takes over work from steroids and can be safely used in the long term. A wonder drug, MMF is also one of the significant treatment components used in patients who receive organ transplants to prevent rejection.

Sister Christy went on MMF for many years without further deterioration. Meanwhile, she was diagnosed with a low-functioning thyroid disease (hypothyroidism) and started on the very safe thyroxine supplementation. But this honeymoon period in her life was relatively short-lived. One day, she unexpectedly developed the same clumsiness in her legs and right hand and suddenly found it difficult to write on or sign papers. The doctors were distraught. She was having a breakthrough of the disease while on treatment at the best possible doses. This meant that her immunosuppression drugs were not maintaining their functions in the long term, and increasing them—even though they would help her gain back functions and reduce symptoms—would also invite severe adverse events. But even then, they did something that every caring doctor would do. They injected her with a high dose of steroids, called pulse therapy, a life-saving intervention in many situations that warrant immediate and urgent immunosuppression. It is safe and was given under monitoring to quickly improve her clinical condition while doctors could usher in other supportive care.

Sister Christy's hands started functioning better two pulses later, and her tremors and clumsiness were gone. But there was something that needed contemplation. A change in her medications was thought out of the box because the MMF had failed. So the physicians treating her decided to bring in the big gun. A drug so powerful that it transforms the immune system ever so gently, like a night-visioned surgical strike on the body without any significant collateral damage. The drug was called rituximab. But rituximab must be used cautiously, as it can reactivate sleeping monsters inside the human body—most importantly, in those who already have weak immune systems, like Sister Christy. She had been under immunosuppression for so long that many hidden terrors within her body would be waiting to wake up once the immune system was hit hard enough for them to reactivate—a condition called emergence of opportunistic infections.

So, before starting rituximab, the doctors screened Sister Christy for hidden viruses and other fungal and bacterial infections to see whether they lay dormant. To their relief, at the baseline, none of these weirdly terrifying infections came back positive. The screening was also performed explicitly for three well-known viruses: HIV, hepatitis B and hepatitis C. A horrific microbe called the JC (John Cunningham) virus—that can worsen brain disease by causing a condition called PML or progressive multifocal leukoencephalopathy, which could kill the patient—was also negative on screening. After ensuring that Sister Christy did not harbour any of these dreadful infections, they initiated her on rituximab.

One week after the rituximab therapy, she felt uneasy, lost her appetite and her abdomen ached. The physicians quickly ran routine diagnostics on her, which showed only one abnormality. She had severe hepatitis.

The treating doctors were flummoxed. They had done everything by the book. Still, Sister Christy landed with a difficult-to-diagnose and unexpected but severe hepatitis. So they checked her for all viruses and resurgence of the autoimmune liver disease again, and none of the testing gave clues or signals as to what was hurting her liver.

There was only one thing to be done. Send her to a place that would get to the bottom of her liver disease, all the while giving her the feeling that she was being protected inside a sanctuary.

So here she was, sitting in front of me, asking for a diagnosis so that she could go back to serving her hospital, her patients and the children she cared for at her residential convent. I looked at waking up an old friend on my journey to help me with the diagnosis of this mysterious severe acute hepatitis that Sister Christy was suffering from: the medical algorithm.

Acute hepatitis has many common causes—from viruses to weird, rare infections by other microbes and even Covid-19. We ruled them out individually until we had no more causes to investigate. However, I kept wondering whether something would have been missed in the clinical history. So I asked the elderly nun about any recent medication changes. Only rituximab was the new drug that was introduced, and she did not use painkillers or over-the-counter medications, and there were no new antibiotics. She categorically denied the use of unscientific and pseudoscientific practices—such as Ayurveda, Siddha and homeopathic remedies—as she did not believe in any such ineffective therapies. There was no other way for us now, and we were left with the only process forward: to ask her liver directly. So I told Sister Christy that we had to biopsy her liver. She was ready for it because her previous doctors had mentioned it would come to this, and that only an expert team could interpret it.

We biopsied her liver. The complexities associated with this case were going way above our heads. We had a patient with a history of autoimmune disease and now new onset severe hepatitis on immunosuppression. None of the viruses had reactivated, and no other cause could be identified. It could never be an autoimmune disease of the liver because Sister Christy was already on treatment for that.

This was medical science. It was factual. It was curious. It had clarity at the beginning and the end. It always found a reason. This clarity can only come when much confusion triggered logic. Here we were, all of us, ultimately waiting for the results of the liver biopsy.

To diagnose Sister Christy.

To get her better.

To get her back home.

Back to her sanctuary, from ours.

I had to do this.

This was personal.

I would give them back what they had given my mother then.

And then I got that call.

The liver biopsy did not show a virus damaging her liver. It did show some mild changes due to autoimmune liver damage. But there was no cancer. There was nothing that was pointing towards an infection. But what it did show was hundreds of peculiar cells that were eating away at the liver, cells called eosinophils. These are usually not expected to be found inside the liver. But they swarm to the liver when there is a special kind of injury.

Drug-induced liver injury.

I slumped back on the chair in front of that microscope.

We had ruled out every drug possible, including alternative medicines that could harm the liver. Sheepishly and with great difficulty, I went back and asked Sister Christy if she was into recreational drugs or other substances of abuse.

I sounded stupid, and she looked calm. 'No,' she answered with composure.

I apologized.

She said she knew what I was doing and that it was not awkward.

She again confirmed her position on all the medications she had taken in the past three months: steroids, rituximab, an occasional medicine for 'gas' and supplements for her bone health because she was on long-term steroids and MMF.

I sat up and asked her, 'What supplements?'

She said they included calcium and vitamin D and a bone-strengthening drug that was very commonly prescribed to those on long-term steroids and immunosuppressants.

My ears sharpened like an elf's as I consumed the information.

'Can you please show me your prescriptions? Every one of them since the last three months?' I asked her.

Sister Christy fished out multiple papers that she had been carrying all the while from a file inside her luggage. I went through document with attentiveness, taking over forty minutes to complete the review of drugs.

Then I found it.

Hiding in plain sight.

~

Salzer and von Baeyer. The lesser-known pharmacists and chemists. The year was 1894. The pharmacist Theodor Salzer described an impurity in phosphoric acid bottles. He called it an impurity and did not bother about it. Two years later, in 1896, an undergraduate student, Hans von Baeyer created an unknown substance. He was at the Royal Academy of Sciences, Munich, Germany, working in the chemical laboratory of his father, Adolf von Baeyer, the winner of the 1905 Nobel Prize in chemistry for discovering the group of chemicals called barbiturates—a category of sedative-hypnotic medications used for treating seizure disorders, anxiety and inducing anaesthesia. Adolf rejected the unknown substance as a 'dreck' or impurity. But young Hans did not let go of his discovery. In 1897, along with his PhD supervisor, Professor Hofmann, he described the synthesis of that compound, later called acetodiphosphoric, which belonged to the group of chemicals called bisphosphonates. However, only after research and development work on these new chemicals by Procter & Gamble (for its detergent uses) was a far more critical action of bisphosphonates unearthed.

These compounds prevented bone resorption—the process in which a substance, such as tissue, is lost by being destroyed and then reabsorbed by the body. Owing to this, they also helped with osteoporosis or thinning of the bones. Chronic use of steroids or immunosuppressants promotes osteoporosis, and most patients are given bisphosphonates as part of the preventive strategy to reduce bone loss and increase strength. However, bisphosphonates have also been linked to severe hepatitis and associated immune-mediated liver injury. This was notable specifically with the compounds zoledronate and ibandronate.

Sister Christy had just received her ibandronate three days before the rituximab injection. Rituximab, per se, was not reported to cause severe hepatitis and could easily be excluded from the list of culprits. Coupled with the finding of the eosinophils on the liver biopsy, and with mild features of autoimmune damage in the absence of every other identifiable cause, the most probable diagnosis for Sister Christy's severe liver injury was the ibandronate that was given to reduce her bone damage. She was restarted on pulsed steroids because it displaced and curbed eosinophil-related liver damage and was quite helpful in this situation. After many days of ordeal, the calm elderly nun's hepatitis resolved, and her energy levels returned.

On the day of discharge, I visited her in the hospital room.

All her bags were packed and she was ready to travel back home.

Sister Christy thanked me as she held my hands tightly, and then she told me, 'Jesus has shown the way; he saved me through you.'

I looked at the other nun, her bystander, and then at Sister Christy again, and smiled at them.

If they wanted to call my science-based medical algorithm 'Jesus', I was okay with that.

As Stephen Hawking said, 'There is a fundamental difference between religion, which is based on authority, [and] science, which is based on observation and reason. Science will win because it works.'

A Diagnosis in 9,46,08,000 Seconds

'Can I play football after the liver transplant?' the sixteen-year-old boy asked me.

'We were told that only you can keep him alive until we find a liver donor,' his frail mother told me.

I psyched myself up with that. Unaware that the three of us would be plunged into battle with a terrifying liver disease and a diagnosis that would take three years to conclude.

~

Three months earlier, Amal was sent home early from school. He complained of severe nausea and fatigue, even vomiting twice, and had a 'bad feeling' while his abdomen groaned with pain. By the end of the week, he was jaundiced, his eyes a deep yellow and urine like he was peeing yellow paint. His legs were swollen, and the abdominal pain worsened. He found sanctuary on his bed and was fatigued most of the time. He was rushed to a nearby clinic and was presumed to have 'mild hepatitis'.

Strangely and unexpectedly, the ultrasound scan of his belly showed features of chronic liver disease, and there was fluid in his abdomen.

The doctors were baffled.

How was that possible? At the age of sixteen, this healthy boy—who did well in school, was active and enjoyed his life—was now suddenly presenting with features of advanced cirrhosis. His liver tests showed high level of jaundice, and other tests showed that his blood was getting thinner, a dangerous finding linked to progressive liver failure.

They referred the boy to the nearest academic hospital because they did not know how to proceed. A group of specialist doctors started working on a diagnosis. Amal underwent a comprehensive clinical history followed by CT scan imaging of the abdomen. Additionally, tests for chronic viral infections, autoimmune liver disease and genetic diseases in children (such as Wilson's disease) were all sent out but came back non-contributory. Given cirrhosis changes on imaging, the presence of portal hypertension (high liver pressures) that resulted in fluid inside his abdomen and liver failure (jaundice, bleeding abnormalities), the doctors decided it was best for Amal to undergo a liver transplantation to sustain life. However, the chances of a transplant were bleak, as a matching donor was not available and the family was not financially stable enough to procure significant funds urgently. The family ran helter-skelter to arrange for funds to realize Amal's life-saving transplantation. His life depended on how fast money could be gathered and not on the quality of the health services available. Nothing else mattered but the money. Meanwhile, he was started on the standard drugs for cirrhosis: diuretic medications, also called water pills, to reduce abdominal fluid; and beta-blocker drugs to reduce liver pressure and prevent massive bleeding.

Amal remained stable for a month. But then, his abdomen started to fill again, and the fluid was accumulating faster than ever—to the point where doctors advised that excess fluid within the abdominal cavity (which was basically fluid that oozed out from the damaged liver surface and lymph channels) had to be removed by inserting a needle and a tube through the abdominal wall and draining it out into a jar. But this proposition was scary for Amal. So he did something that would take care of the fluid slowly but efficiently—he stopped taking salt in his diet. Restricting sodium reduces fluid accumulation in patients with cirrhosis. This worked well for Amal, but then he started losing interest in food because the dishes were tasteless, and eating became a chore. He lost a lot of weight and muscle in the process. He was getting malnourished. As his condition grew from stable to worse, it was then that they searched for a second opinion to fall back onto something more hopeful. Liver transplantation was becoming a pipe dream.

So here they were, mother and son, with folded hands, asking me to help them understand what was hurting Amal's liver. A thorough evaluation of the previous tests was performed at our unit. Everything was fitting with cirrhosis and high-liver-pressure-related complications.

But what was causing it? Everyone seemed to have left this question flaccid. There had to be something that everyone had missed.

In the months preceding the onset of symptoms, the use of liver-toxic drugs and Ayurvedic and other herbal medications were denied. Unusually, the swelling on the legs looked disproportionate to the swelling of the abdomen. This was very peculiar because in cirrhosis, the swelling due to fluid build-up was supposed to be predominant in the abdomen and unlikely in the legs. But this could happen in one condition: a rare disease called Budd Chiari Syndrome or BCS.

In this disease, the abdomen and legs swell up when there is a block in a large vein of the abdomen (called inferior vena cava or IVC) or the veins inside the liver (hepatic veins, which take out blood from the liver to the heart through the IVC). So we looked at the CT imaging again and were more attentive this time. The IVC vein was fine, and so were the hepatic veins, and classical features such as large, tortuous veins over the abdomen (collaterals) and inside the gastrointestinal tract (varices)—usually notable in patients with BCS—were absent in Amal. Thus, BCS was effectively ruled out.

We looked at other rare causes for cirrhosis in a child, and none showed up on the tests we so carefully chose and performed. Exhausting every single option, we were left with nothing other than the liver biopsy. But we were unsure what we were looking for; we were travelling the path that the medical algorithm took us. But a biopsy was not easy in the presence of abdominal fluid; due to the high risk of bleeding, the little piece of tissue had to be taken safely from Amal's liver. We performed the transjugular liver biopsy. It was like an angiography procedure, and Amal tolerated it well. The biopsy reports were expedited. But the results did not help us much except one happy little finding: there was no cirrhosis. Amal's liver was not affected by chronic liver disease as was previously thought. Everyone was astonished.

The liver-biopsy findings were the strangest. In a few scattered areas, the blood channels within the liver (sinusoids) were dilated.

But the even stranger finding was the presence of a peculiar type of scarring (fibrosis) of the liver tissue around the sinusoids—known as perisinusoidal fibrosis. This was a non-specific finding notable in the progression of liver disease leading to cirrhosis—a cause for the same cannot be identified solely based on its presence on a liver-biopsy sample. Classically called 'chicken wire fibrosis', it is associated with severe fatty liver disease. However, the only issue here was that this boy's liver tissue lacked fat deposits, and the peculiar scarring was not related to fatty liver disease. Perisinusoidal scarring can be seen rarely in non-cirrhotic portal hypertension or NCPH. As you may recall from the case of our patient Suresh, NCPH is a group of liver disorders in which clinical features of increased liver pressures existed in the absence of chronic liver disease or cirrhosis.

We found a scientifically peer-reviewed published paper from 1979 on it! However, Amal's profile did not fit the clinical picture that the authors described, even though we did not have any diagnosis to offer other than NCPH of the perisinusoidal fibrosis variety. The biopsy report was bittersweet for all of us. Sweet because there was no cirrhosis, and bitter since Amal remained undiagnosed. I was not satisfied. But we had nothing more to do. Amal was getting better, and once the abdominal fluid was gone, he started gaining his appetite and his hopes returned. He started performing activities independently and the jaundice resolved slowly and steadily. We were all just happy for him, and I was delighted too; even without a working and realistic diagnosis, if the young patient was getting better, then that was all that was needed to make the journey worthwhile. Sometimes, a happy patient was enough. Things looked fine, and Amal and his mother thanked us because they could avoid a transplant. There was no permanent damage to the liver, and we all looked at it as some 'unknown acute insult' that led to 'perisinusoidal fibrosis' and portal hypertension, which resolved in due course.

I remembered these words by Voltaire: 'The art of medicine consists of amusing the patient while nature cures the disease.'

While many things in healthcare cannot be explained immediately, all things have an explanation. We could not figure this one out, but we left it alone because the patient had improved.

Back home, when I slept or at dinner with my wife and my children, these words would echo spontaneously and without warning:

Can I play football after the liver transplant?

We were told that only you can keep him alive until we find a donor.

Something in me yearned for more answers.

I felt incomplete, and this worried me.

Something sinister was coming to haunt me, and I could feel it in my bones. Something was hiding, waiting to strike. Something terrible.

I pushed away these feelings and covered them up with the sweet casings that everyday life gave me from being with my family. Delightful memories took over my dreadful premonitions.

I did not hear from Amal or his mother for almost two years, and the sinister feeling passed. The past was buried.

I shifted to a new hospital and started at a new clinical unit, leaving behind my old practice and office.

~

One fine day in 2019, I was called to the emergency room to see a sick boy.

He was eighteen years old.

As I walked down the stairs leading to the triage room, that sinister feeling—a worry of doom, that terrifying intuition that I felt years ago after bidding goodbye to Amal and his mother—came back without warning.

I stopped midway to catch my breath and calm my mind, and then I saw him.

Can I play football after the liver transplant?

I saw Amal on that emergency room triage bed, gasping for breath, his abdomen distended and fluid-filled. They had travelled six hours by road to reach where I was.

Amal's mother was missing, but his uncle was here this time.

I asked the elderly man, 'What has been happening?'

He told me that everything was fine until two months ago. But then, one day, Amal started feeling tired. His legs got progressively swollen, and the abdomen distended with fluid, which had worsened during the past three weeks. They were unsure where to find me because I had left the previous hospital and they could not trace me. Amal had started to restrict salt and found that his swelling reduced. He had followed my years-old advice to stabilize himself, but he could barely manage. He then saw the details of my new place from a YouTube video that I had made and asked his uncle to bring him to where I was now. I was at a faraway place, but for Amal, this was the place he wanted to be. As he told me, when it was a bad day, inside that darkness, my face was the only one he remembered. He trusted me because I kept my word the last time he had come in critically ill. I had kept him alive, and he went back to playing football.

My heart sank as I looked at Amal, and I closed my eyes and wondered at the power of this disease. Whatever it was, I knew it was going to beat me, beat all of us. It would put me in my place and make me understand that doctors were human and helpless. In my mind, I kept replaying Amal's death on a ventilator. First, I had to convince myself that this was a terrifying battle and that I had to be ready to lose. Only when I had accepted that fact could I make the family receptive to the truth of incoming death, about someone gone too soon. I spoke to Amal, and he was oriented and aware of everything I had said. I told him that we had to drain the fluid in his belly and that even though he was scared, it would help him breathe well. And he concurred. We drained the ascites—the massively collected abdominal fluid inside Amal—and stabilized him over the next few hours.

I wanted to know what was happening to him.

I tried to understand that which was beating us at every step.

Hiding for years and then killing Amal slowly.

I wasted no time, and a second liver biopsy was planned. Whatever was killing Amal's liver was a disease so sinister that it had evolved over years to strike fatally. Blood tests and imaging would not help us get to the bottom of this enigmatic illness. However, Amal and his family did not have money to afford another transjugular biopsy. After much begging and debating with the management, we got it done for free. Amal went through it without any significant events and was shifted to the ICU for observation.

But the fluid in his abdomen was slowly re-accumulating.

One late evening, as I was about to leave my outpatient department, I got a call from my pathologist. She told me the words I was waiting to hear for almost two years: 'We got it.'

I sat on my chair, exhaled and heaved a sigh of relief.

'But,' she said, 'I have compared it with his previous liver biopsy, and now it seems like Amal has developed cirrhosis.'

The news was not good. Not good at all.

A liver disease progressing to cirrhosis in a matter of two years?

I was terrified and troubled.

Usually, it takes decades for cirrhosis to develop. In Amal, it was lightning-fast.

But there were exceptions. Certain conditions could trigger liver injury so overwhelming, that chronic liver damage and cirrhosis could set in quickly, within a few years.

Amal was harbouring one such disease.

~

Veno-occlusive disease or VOD (now SOS, as mentioned earlier) is a terrifying, rare disease of the liver usually seen in bone marrow transplant recipients and in patients receiving chemotherapy and radiation treatments. This dreadful disease could also occur with the use of certain drugs and toxins. We saw it in our patient Deepak earlier in the chapter, as you may recall. In this disease, the blood cells lining the liver cells, called the sinusoidal endothelial, experience damage from the exposure of certain toxic metabolites. In the early stages, the disease may not fully manifest, and the findings occur in a scattered pattern that may be wholly missed on the liver biopsy.

Clinically, in the early phase, patients may present with only lower limb swelling and abdominal fluid collection, or generalized body swelling, depending on the severity of liver injury. Over a few weeks, the inflammation and scar tissue thicken in and around the affected blood vessels inside the liver, leading to dense scarring that later evolves into cirrhosis. Amal's history was devoid of drugs and toxins—two most common causes for severe SOS in liver.

But we had to be sure.

We asked his uncle again regarding the use of drugs or supplements long back, to the time when I first met Amal all those years ago. Alternative medicines, supplements and everything we could think of, including folk medicine use. We kept asking him leading questions.

And this time, we clinched it.

Something we had missed so long back, but now it had surfaced.

One month before his initial presentation, Amal was diagnosed with a condition called protein-losing enteropathy—a condition in which proteins are lost in the faeces due to a structural change in the intestines. In Amal, the protein loss was diagnosed as secondary to a different condition called small intestinal lymphangiectasia, in which abnormal lymph channels dilate on the walls of the intestines and ooze protein-rich fluid into the gut. The fluid secreted by these lymph channels, rich in protein, was getting lost in Amal's stools. This resulted in lower-limb swelling due to protein loss. The gastroenterologist who saw Amal at the time advised only follow-up, a protein-rich diet and some medications to reduce swelling as he needed them, but not daily. However, the leg swelling was causing Amal trouble while playing football, and his uncle had taken him to a local traditional healer—an 'expert' in treating such swellings of the leg—who gave Amal a mixture of herbs to 'cure' his illness. Amal took the herbs for close to two weeks, and a week later, he started developing symptoms that resulted in his initial clinical deterioration. His mother did not feel the need to disclose this at the time, since she would have thought that herbal supplements and traditional medical practices were perfectly safe because they were natural.

I asked Amal's uncle, 'Do you remember the name of the herbs?'

And he said, 'Yes, in Malayalam language, it is called kilukilukki.'

This herb was locally known as 'baby's rattle' and commonly as 'rattle-weed'. It belongs to the family of plants known as crotalaria, so called because the dry pods make the sound of a rattle when shaken. In traditional medicine, this plant was used to treat urinary symptoms and fever; a poultice of the roots was commonly applied to swollen joints to reduce inflammation; or extracts were consumed to dispel intestinal worms. The folk healer thought Amal's leg swelling was due to a group of worms called 'filaria' and prescribed him extracts of rattlepod leaves for consumption to treat it.

However, the fact was that the crotalaria group of plants were very toxic to the liver because they contained pyrrolizidine alkaloids, which are strongly associated with the dreadful disease SOS. Amal had developed crotalaria-induced liver injury, which started as a limited and focal SOS disease in the liver, but soon steadily and silently progressed to full-blown cirrhosis secondary to chronic SOS.

The prognosis was terrible because there was no way to stop or reverse that injury. This was not like the first time Amal had met me. In this precarious situation, he needed a liver transplantation to survive. The only drug that was recommended for the treatment of SOS, called defibrotide, was not available in India at the time and was too expensive for Amal's family to afford. Moreover, like before, there was no donor and no funding. But after restarting the water pills, Amal's swelling resolved, and he clinically became a little better. But we still had that cirrhosis to deal with. After extensively discussing options with the family, we thought we would do something out of the box.

In 2014, a group of researchers from the University of Guadalajara treated patients with chronic hepatitis C infection and advanced fibrosis (liver scarring) with a drug called pirfenidone, which was special. Scientists found that pirfenidone reduced scarring and improved liver regeneration in those with symptoms due to chronic viral infection. This drug was called an 'anti-fibrotic'. We had no other options. Amal and his family had none either. After completing the process of informed consent, we put Amal on pirfenidone and followed up for one whole year. A third liver biopsy was taken once the period of treatment was over, and we were astonished. The scars in the liver had almost dissolved, and the normal liver tissue was regenerating inside Amal. His cirrhosis was getting reversed. Something everyone had difficulty in accepting.

But it was real.

The findings under the microscope were proof.

After almost two years of treatment, Amal stopped taking pirfenidone because his liver imaging did not show features of cirrhosis or its progression.

We published Amal's story in a peer-reviewed publication in 2019.

Since 2022, Amal has not visited me in my outpatient department for any complications related to his liver disease. But he still messages me on WhatsApp, and he likes my family's photos on Instagram, where he follows me.

And he still plays football.

That is how I know we did okay.

It is not the medical books that teach us real clinical medicine—it is the patients. The more you care for them, the more you will learn to beat the odds.

Killing Me Softly

'I feel like killing myself,' the elderly man told me. He was gloomy, and his life burdensome.

'I cannot sleep. I have not slept for days and nights. I am disoriented in the morning,' he continued. 'There is no place that comforts me. I was told that I would find answers here. Could you please help me? Free me from this terrible itching.'

I sat face to face with the man who was profoundly jaundiced and itching terribly all over his body. He used a sharp wooden contraption, one that gnawed into his skin, to itch hard-to-reach places. His skin was dry, and there were bleeding spots, but he scratched through it all. Some areas were infected, but the scratching did not dent the itching feeling. He remained unsatisfied, however much he continued abrading his skin. I readied myself to face this agonizing liver disease that had demonically possessed this man's life.

He was suffering from a condition called cholestatic hepatitis, the reasons for which remained unknown.

We were his last hope. The final frontier.

~

A month earlier, the old man, Haneefa, started to lose his appetite. Routine chores and walks felt draining. He lost energy. A week after his troubles began, he noticed his palms and soles were itchy. At first, he shook it off, thinking they were allergies. But as days went by, he noticed that his urine was darkly coloured, and then the whites (sclera) of his eyes started to turn yellow (scleral icterus). These were the signs and symptoms of jaundice. As the jaundice worsened, so did the itching, which was now all over his body. The more he scratched, the worse it got.

Days and nights went by, with lost sleep and deepening jaundice. The lack of sleep made him groggy the next day, and his mental health suffered progressively. He would tip and fall, move around like a zombie, a true embodiment of *The Walking Dead*. He went to a nearby drug store, where the pharmacist gave him a drug called cetirizine for the itching. It did not help at all. He stayed alone. His wife had died a few years ago.

When he realized it was not just an 'allergy' and would not go away, he reached out for help. He called his son, who was working and living far away. A day later, his son, Basheer, came home to a shocking surprise. The jaundice on his father's face struck him first, then the skin changes. His father was using forks and tree branches to scratch where it itched the worst, and his skin had peeled off, blistering and bleeding in places. Something was incredibly wrong.

In a record amount of time, Haneefa was admitted to the ward of a nearby multispeciality hospital the same day. The doctors started evaluating him without delay. The liver test results were through the roof. High bilirubin, raised liver enzymes, predominantly ALP and GGT. Jaundice and itching (called pruritus in medical terms) in a person is always, at first, suspected to be of cholestatic type until proven otherwise.

Cholestatic jaundice, or obstructive jaundice, is a condition in which bile flow is either hampered at the liver cell or bile duct level (within the ducts inside or outside the liver), resulting in stagnation of bile and build-up of bile acids in the blood, which causes severe itching. Haneefa's high liver enzymes showed that this wasn't just a 'block' in the flow of bile. It was *cholestatic hepatitis*. The whole machinery itself was under attack: Both the liver cells (hepatocytes) and the bile system cells (cholangiocytes) were inflamed. In general, cholestatic jaundice can be due to diseases at the liver-cell level (intrahepatic-hepatocellular cholestasis), bile ducts within the liver (intrahepatic-biliary cholestasis) or bile ducts outside the liver (post-hepatic or extrahepatic cholestasis). With this general idea of symptoms and signs, the doctors treating Haneefa initiated tests for suspected causes. The ultrasound, CT scans and MRCP (MRI of the bile ducts inside and outside the liver) did not show blocks to bile drainage. This essentially meant that all tumours, duct stones and duct strictures (narrowing of ducts) inside and outside the liver were ruled out.

The physicians then pondered these test results. This meant that Haneefa had cholestatic jaundice and hepatitis, which was not due to an obstructive cause (old term: 'surgical jaundice'). If obstructive causes were ruled out, it was time to look at causes that damaged the liver (hepatocellular) and bile duct cells (cholangiocyte) within the organ. Infections, including viruses and parasites; alcohol use; diseases affecting the blood vessels in the liver; genetic causes that affected the liver, especially those that caused bile stagnation in adults; and bile duct diseases, such as primary biliary cholangitis and primary sclerosing cholangitis, were all effectively ruled out.

So they were left with an essential cause of cholestatic hepatitis: drugs or medications, including anabolic steroids. However, Haneefa denied any medication use and did not consume any over-the-counter herbal or non-herbal dietary pills or supplements. The doctors were stumped. They were focused on treating his symptoms rather than the cause(s) for those symptoms, as they got more clarity on the now enigmatic diagnosis. Steroids were started to reduce liver inflammation and jaundice, which was standard practice in such cases when several infections, tumours or blocks were not identified. Alongside the steroids, the primary drug to reduce itching was given—known as ursodeoxycholic acid, or UDCA, at doses of 10–15 mg/kg body weight. It worked for a while, with Haneefa's itching largely reducing. But the jaundice and liver-enzyme levels were slowly but persistently increasing.

Five days after treatment initiation, Haneefa improved marginally, but his general condition worsened. He started having suicidal thoughts because the lack of sleep gave him a thundering headache, and his whole body felt as if it was being pelted with large stones and burned at the stake. His skin blistered and oozed, as the itching was relentless. When the situation got out of hand, the doctors advised Basheer to take his father to a specialized liver disease unit. Travelling more than 300 kilometres, the good son brought his now nearly suicidal father to our department for further care.

~

One look at Haneefa, and we knew something was off. Something sinister had followed him, avoiding us, lurking in the shadows of a mysterious diagnosis, waiting to strike. The cholestatic hepatitis was so severe that his liver functions were deteriorating rapidly. But there was a thumb rule in cholestatic hepatitis, and we hoped that would come true in Haneefa's case too. That would give us ample time to figure out the cause of the man's troubling illness. The realistic chances that a patient developed liver failure were far less with the cholestatic type of liver injury compared to acute hepatitis.

None of the drug treatments were improving Haneefa's itching. He had requested only one thing from us: to help him sleep well for at least one night. In severe cholestasis, when drugs do not work, therapeutic plasma exchange, or TPE, is the last option left to reduce the itching. As we know, in TPE, the 'bad' plasma from the blood is removed and replaced with freshly thawed, healthy donor plasma to reduce the levels of circulating toxins and bile acids responsible for the severe itch. The process also does something else for cholestasis patients. It reduces the high levels of bilirubin responsible for the jaundice. So we started Haneefa on TPE, since the first and only request that the patient had was that we improve his symptoms and give him comfort. The diagnosis could wait.

All patients do not come out of a textbook. In real life, one must first centralize patient needs. An ideal scenario would be that the doctor caters to patient care and addresses concerns rather than initiates an investigation spree from the word go. After three quick sessions of TPE, Haneefa saw substantial improvement in his symptoms. After more than two weeks, when the TPE sessions improved symptoms so much that he finally experienced a good night's sleep, Haneefa was more open to discussions about causes. It was time to really start probing that place where we would find real answers to his mysterious cholestatic hepatitis. It was not within reports. Not within scanned images. Not within other doctors' notes. But in asking the patient himself for a diagnosis.

Clinical history is the most crucial powerhouse of a medicine tool for identifying a mysterious diagnosis. Hippocrates once said, 'It was more important to know what sort of person had the disease than to know what sort of disease the person had.'

With Haneefa, we saw, heard, listened, spoke and went through every aspect of his clinical history and ruled out every clue that linked hepatitis to infection, cancer, drugs or supplements. But then, something my colleague saw on the chart prompted another round of clinically relevant investigation of his history. Haneefa's blood marker for control of blood sugars (glucose), an indicator of reasonable diabetes control, was relatively high; his glycated haemoglobin, HbA1c, was 9.2 per cent. This meant that Haneefa had diabetes, and if he knew it, he had to be on medications for the same.

'What medicines were you taking for diabetes?' my colleague asked.

'None, sir,' came the reply. 'I was on only complete diet management.'

'What kind of diet?' was our leading question.

'An Ayurvedic practitioner advised me, and I followed that. No medicines and no supplements, but only natural measures.'

'What all did it include?' we probed further.

'He mostly advised me to follow a highly restricted vegetarian diet but asked me to add a special dried and powdered plant during each meal.'

We sat up, all our antennas sharpened, as we asked him to describe the powder and its contents. There were no contents, only one ingredient, a herb that Haneefa dried, powdered and consumed. He showed us a picture of it on his phone, then proceeded to tell us what it contained.

Gymnema sylvestre is a woody vine native to Asia. It is called 'madhunashini' or 'sugar destroyer' in ancient Ayurvedic texts, and was used traditionally for controlling diabetes and for weight loss in the form of gymnema teas. However, there was no good evidence that any of the promoted claims were true. Pre-clinical studies showed some effects of sugar-lowering with gymnema, but none were proven through rigorous clinical trials in humans. The mechanism of action of gymnema was also mostly based on 'assumptions' and had no realistically proven effects in humans.

An interesting finding was that the gymnema plant chemicals, gurmarin and gymnemic acids, blunted human taste buds towards sweet and bitters. This resulted in lower food intake, which reduced overall calorie intake, indirectly, and arguably represented the possible 'good control' of diabetes associated with potential weight loss. Some peer-reviewed published studies showed that people refused to eat candies after being given gymnema extracts! But there was another side to the gymnema story—the plant chemicals were potentially liver toxic, and emerging reports suggested that it could cause cholestatic hepatitis.

Once we ruled out all other competing causes, using unique methods utilized for the diagnosis of herb-induced liver injury (known as causality assessment tools), gymnema was found to be the culprit for Haneefa's prolonged and mysterious cholestatic hepatitis. We were glad we could finally diagnose him. We proved this by subjecting Haneefa to a much-awaited liver biopsy, which showed classical features of such an injury to liver cells and bile duct cells, leading to a block in bile flow at both the liver- and the bile-duct-cell level—intrahepatic biliary cholestasis! After almost a month and a half in our hospital, and on close follow-up, there was finally a complete resolution of Haneefa's hepatitis. During the last follow-up, he bade us all farewell. He held my hand tight and told me he wanted to see me occasionally—as a friend and not as a doctor—and I concurred.

But there was something about that handshake and that hold, and I felt as if he was holding on to me. As if it was not the end, and I would see him again. A dark cloud loomed inside my room. Before he left, I told Haneefa to check his liver tests every one or two months, just to be sure. He nodded and walked out of my room.

Intuition: the ability to understand something instinctively without needing conscious reasoning.

A significant part of clinical medicine is intuition.

It comes with seeing many patients. Treating many more. Saving some, losing others and helping a lot of them. It helps a doctor find sanctuary for a patient that approaches him. It helps him outline the boundaries of that sanctuary. But then some diseases do not play by the rules. A doctor must never put his guard down. An evolving symptom or a sign, and complications that lay low, emerge only to overwhelm later, without warning.

This is what makes a doctor human. The same insecurities and worries that plague the patient become theirs.

I've learnt that no matter how much knowledge or experience I gather, I am still helpless at times. There will be moments I lose, even after doing everything right. I've come to accept that truth. Being a doctor is not about winning—it's about being there when it matters most.

~

Four months passed by, and I got no call from or news about Haneefa, and he comfortably went into a corner of my heart where I made sanctuary for him. But then one day, unexpectedly, when everything remained forgotten, I got a call from my emergency physician about a prior patient who was sick and wanted to see me as soon as possible. I walked into the emergency bay to see Haneefa on a trolley and his son nearby. Deeply worried, his son told me that his father had been doing well all these months, but for one week, he had stopped eating and had been 'growing thin'. His diabetes was well controlled because he had moved on to insulin and stopped all kinds of herbal and supplement treatment, but his blood tests, done at a hospital near their home, were profoundly worrying.

I looked at Haneefa and saw that his eyes were not as deep a yellow as when I first met him. But his liver tests showed severe hepatitis—his enzymes were again through the roof, but without jaundice. And something else, something unexpected, was happening: his white cell counts, haemoglobin, platelets, all of them were dropping rapidly. The haematologist, a specialist in blood disorders, was called in. After sending relevant baseline tests, he ordered an immediate bone marrow examination. The bone marrow aspiration and biopsy were performed and the pathologist quickly reviewed it for an early provisional report.

To our great dismay and surprise, the bone marrow tests showed something sinister, and we were stumped. Haneefa's bone marrow was failing, and because of that, his blood counts were dropping: a condition called aplastic anaemia. We were now back to figuring out the reason for his newly diagnosed mystery illness. Was this related to his previous liver disease, or was something else causing the aplastic anaemia?

Multiple factors can cause aplastic anaemia. With great difficulty, a lot more investigations and after many sleepless nights we ruled out every possible cause we could test for. Finally, we were left with a last cause, one that the medical community woefully and foolishly considered when there was no hope and reason. A diagnosis termed 'idiopathic', which meant 'that which remains unknown'—a term I hate from the bottom of my heart in clinical medicine. Nothing in scientific medicine is idiopathic. Everything that happened had to happen for a reason, an underlying cause. Clinical medicine is our playground. Our rules, our game. We live and die on this hill. I would never let a patient go without knowing what was hurting them, gnawing at them.

Everything in Haneefa fit into the 'idiopathic' designation—except one thing. The hepatitis—it was back, without jaundice but with aplastic anaemia. So we searched the literature and came face to face with a new kind of monster. Something we never knew about, a diagnosis that I had never heard of before, but one that was real and so sinister that it had killed every patient that it became the diagnosis of.

'H triple A' or 'HAAA', also known as hepatitis-associated aplastic anaemia. There was only one intervention that could save Haneefa's life: a salvage bone marrow transplantation. Our unit, at the time, did not have one, and so Haneefa was emergently referred for a matching workup and bone marrow transplant to the nearest specialized centre. As he was rolled out of the ICU, he held my hand and asked me if he could come back to me for a follow-up because his confidence and zest to live existed only in my presence. When he shook my hands, as if he was 'holding on', I thought deeply and told him that we would meet again, and that I would continue to care for him.

But my vulnerable mind, lost in chaos at the time, was telling me otherwise. This would be the last time I would see Haneefa, touch him or speak to him. However, human nature is resilient. I fought the evil thought and hoped to see him again, to serve him. The worst part of having a patient diagnosed with aplastic anaemia is that you do not get time to work for them—the disease is cunningly relentless, and it destroys every little type of blood cell. This made the patient prone to a host of life-threatening infections, a ruleless playground for microbes, and it was only a matter of time before multiple organ failures set in.

Five days after I last saw Haneefa, I got a call from Basheer. *Some good news at last,* I thought. Maybe they got a matching donor and everything was fine. Everything had to be because we were right in our diagnosis, we got it in time and were on time to transfer him out for the best care.

The first words I heard were, 'Doctor, thank you,'—and my heart swelled because I felt the hope … but they were followed by the shattering words that killed my hope.

Haneefa was no more. During the workup for bone marrow transplant and donor fitness, he developed a severe fungal infection that spilled into his bloodstream, rapidly reaching and damaging his brain and lungs. Since no medications that they gave helped him improve blood counts, his body withered away trying to fight a monstrous infection in the absence of a functioning immune system. He had been on the ventilator due to multiple organ failure and died of severe fungal infection.

I kept the phone down and sat in my chair for a while, numb from the loss of my patient. Numb from understanding that medicine was all about trying by stretching your limits, but still, at times, failing dishearteningly. In medicine, we learn something new every day, always the hard way. We were the first to identify that herbal medicines can cause hepatitis, followed by the devastating HAAA syndrome, leading to death. We published our findings in a scientific journal after a peer review so that every physician who read it would know that the use of the gymnema herb, and possibly other herbs like it, could be deadly.

What if Haneefa had not been scared of scientifically tested drugs?

What if he had been on insulin?

What if there had been no alternative medicine practitioners in this story?

I would never have met Haneefa.

He would be alive.

He would have been playing with his grandchildren someday in the future.

But I was thankful.

Thankful that I got the opportunity to serve him in his darkest days.

Thankful to be there on that journey, even though it messed me up and gave me scars.

I will carry them to my grave.

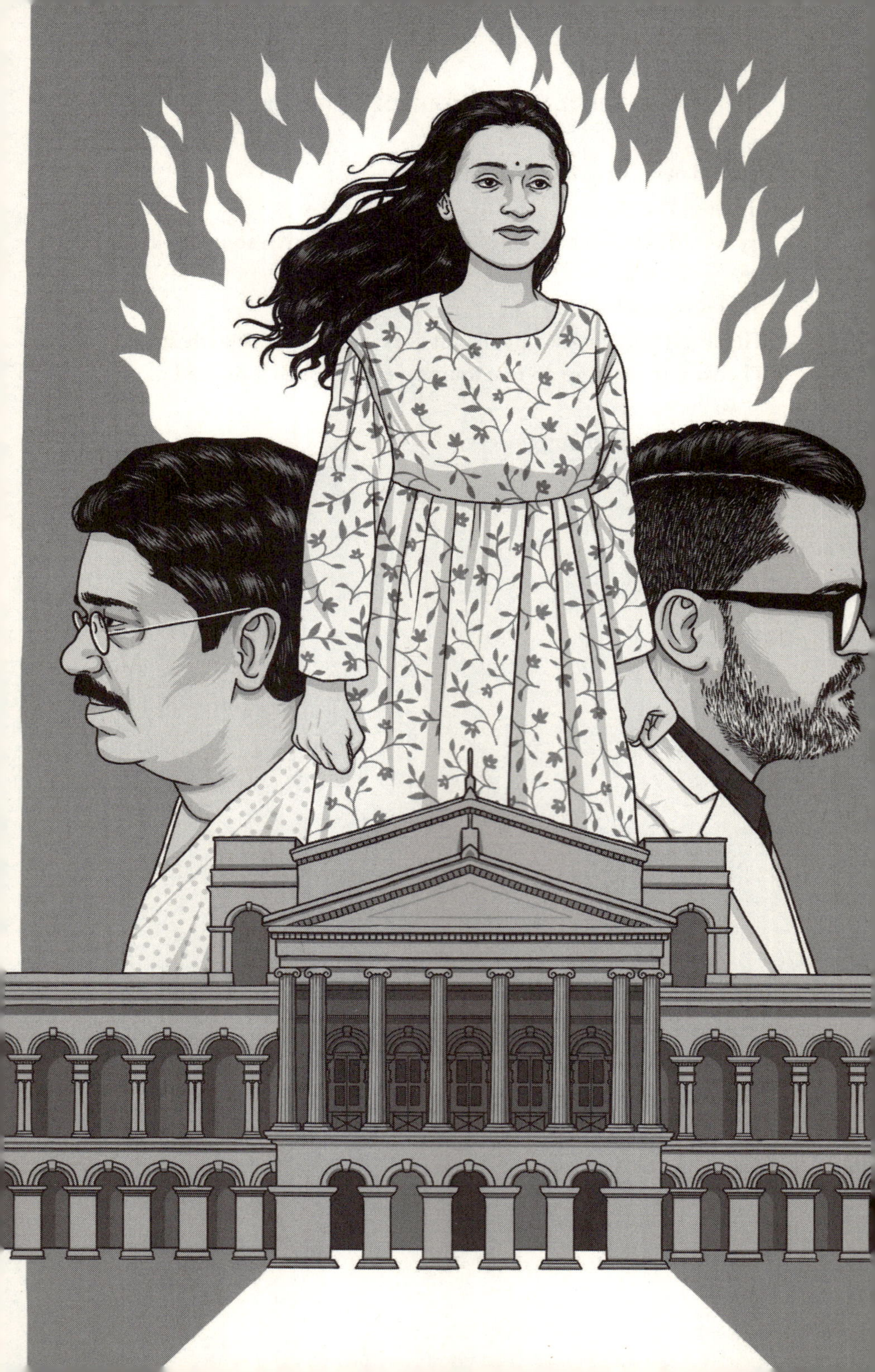

CHAPTER 10

When the Crabs Come Marching to Eden

Confrontations and Negotiations with Liver Cancer and Other Such Dread

The Conqueror Gift

'Don't limit your challenges, challenge your limits.'
—Unknown

I met Ratheesh in October 2022. He wanted to know if he could survive his liver failure on medications alone. But there was more than met the eye with his case, and I found something else, greatly sinister, haunting him and slowly eating away from the inside.

What followed was an intense battle against not one but two terrifying foes.

Cancer.

And time.

And a unique love story that conquered both.

Ratheesh's family was small but big at heart—very close-knit, with a loving father, a daughter and a mother who bound them all in the deepest fondness. After a brief infection that everyone thought was benign and passing, Ratheesh found himself looking at the deep yellowness in his eyes. In a few days, he found himself in a precarious position. He was diagnosed at his nearby clinic with jaundice, and the reason was a failing liver due to cirrhosis or chronic liver damage. As you may recall from earlier discussions, in cirrhosis, the liver undergoes scarring and shrinkage. Along with it, the liver pressures rise, leading to a host of complications. Cirrhosis is a terrible disease. As scarring progresses, along with the liver failure, multiple other complications take shape. This is heralded by jaundice, followed by the failure of different organ systems, such as the brain, kidney, lungs and heart. The organ failure does not follow any specific order. One day, a patient could be well, and the next day, he could be on dialysis, while another would be in a coma on the ventilator.

The mere presence of liver failure thrust the patient into days of unexpected complications—some so terrible that family members often developed post-traumatic stress disorder seeing the patient go through such ravaging clinical events. It was akin to bogeys of a never-ending train that kept crashing on you.

There are five stages in cirrhosis. But there is also a sixth one, a point of no return that usually ends in death. These are known as the Baveno stages, named after a small lakeside town in Italy. The town was made famous by a niche group of liver specialists who devised a team to develop universal guidelines for physicians caring for liver patients to treat cirrhosis and its complications predictably. The group's first meeting was not in Baveno but in Groningen, in the Netherlands, led by the late Professor Andrew Burroughs in 1986. It was the second meeting that was conducted at the lakeside town of Baveno. They called it Baveno I, and it changed everything we knew about liver disease management in the current era. The Baveno I conference was headed by Professor Roberto de Franchis, a prominent clinical scientist. It also featured Professor Roberto Grossmann—another global leader and pillar of hepatology. His studies on liver pressures led to the discovery of beta-blocker drugs as a treatment to reduce portal-hypertension-related complications by another stalwart of hepatology, Professor Didier Lebrec from France.

I was part of Baveno 6, as my mentor gave me that opportunity. My professor and teacher, Dr Shiv Kumar Sarin, is one among the last original pillars of hepatology that remain today. In Baveno, I felt tiny and saw far on the shoulders of giants.

It was the Baveno group that described with clarity and endorsed the five stages that patients with cirrhosis go through. The old staging, called the Child–Pugh class, was no longer essential. It was far easier to discuss treatments based on the Baveno staging. Patients who were persistently in Stage 4 or who moved to Stage 5 had one option for cure: a liver transplant. Baveno Stage 5 was when jaundice entered the natural history of the disease. It meant that the liver was failing, and there was very little time left for the patient in this world. However, it was not the Baveno group that initially described the stages. They endorsed it from someone else's original work.

In 2014, Gennaro D'Amico and his colleagues first described the stage-wise progression that defined the natural history of cirrhosis, making it easy to understand how cirrhosis patients behaved with every complication that burdened them. A robust, predictive clinical tool was born.

When doctors who first evaluated Ratheesh saw his blood tests, they immediately knew that he had very little time left. He was in Stage 5—he had skipped the progression from each stage. But they were confused about why this had happened. Ratheesh was advised to get reviewed at a specialist centre for better advice and deeper evaluation. So here he was in front of me, wanting to know if he could survive the dreadful Stage 5 on medications alone. He could, if we could find a reversible cause for his liver failure and treat it. Treating the cause of such rapid progression, once reversible, would help Ratheesh come down to Stage 2 and save him from an immediate, mandated liver transplantation.

Unfortunately, an infection had worsened his previously undiagnosed liver cirrhosis. But even after that infection had passed, Ratheesh did not improve to a lower stage. There was something else lurking in the dark that was opportunistically hurting his liver, and we had to figure it out. And fast.

Ratheesh underwent focused tests at our centre, and the reason why he did not improve slowly came to light. Within that shrunken, failing liver was a giant tumour. A liver cancer was eating Ratheesh's liver from the inside, worsening its function and making it impossible for it to recover to the lower stages. We were left with not one but two challenges.

A failing liver. And a cancer inside the failing liver.

To treat cancer of the liver, or hepatocellular carcinoma (HCC), we looked at the work of another group that changed the way we treated cancer of the liver. The BCLC strategy, also called the Barcelona Clinic Liver Cancer group strategy. The BCLC made an algorithm to provide the best treatment options for patients with cirrhosis suffering from liver cancer, the BCLC staging. There were five stages: 0 and A to D, with D being the worst. In Stage D, the expected survival was only three months. Ratheesh was in Stage D because he had liver failure along with cancer. Early treatment options—such as burning the tumour from the outside (RFA or MWA; using radiofrequencies or microwaves to destroy cancer) or from the inside (TACE, which involved a small dose of chemotherapy agent; or TARE, in which liquid containing radioactive mini-beads were explicitly injected into the blood vessel supplying the tumour to kill it from within [out of the question in the presence of jaundice])—were deemed unsafe in Stage D. We could not let Ratheesh die.

Even though Baveno's strategy told us that patients with liver failure and liver cancer required only the best supportive care and end-of-life care until death, this was not a realistic option for us. Ratheesh was only forty-eight years old, and his tumour was not very aggressive. It had not spread out of the liver and did not locally advance inside the liver, as in Stage C. He was not bedridden and was not critically ill. Yet. Ratheesh was among a special group of patients who still had the option of life-saving transplantation even at the end stages of liver cancer, as per criteria—a BCLC strategy exception.

I told Ratheesh that medicines could never save him.

It had to be a liver transplant. He had three months left.

The end of February in 2023 would be the most likely time he would die without a transplant.

This was etched in stone.

They had no money, and they had no matching donors. Hearing about his plight, distant relatives came forward as potential donors. All were rejected because they did not match as expected. Ratheesh was then put on the brain-dead liver donor (the deceased liver-donation programme) list under the state-government-run programme. But voluntary organ donations did not come as expected. If they did come, it was purely by chance.

While he was waiting for a liver donor, something else entered our well-laid-out plan. Baveno Stage 6. The guidelines do not mention it. But it was real, and it was terrifying. It was the harbinger of death. And without warning, who we believed was a stable patient, Ratheesh, entered our ICU, fighting for his life as another bout of severe infection destroyed all hope. The biggest foe that patients with cirrhosis faced was an unexpected infection. It could be a passing flu or a life-threatening blood infection.

~

It was December 2022, and there were no matching living donors or voluntary brain-dead donor livers in sight. One morning, Ratheesh felt breathless and giddy. He lost his balance as well as his mind. He mumbled and fumbled and got so sick that when he landed in the emergency department, his blood pressure was so low and his pulse so weak that large boluses of fluid had to be pushed into him to get his heart to beat stronger. He was in a condition called sepsis, in which an infection resulted in at least one organ failure. Sometimes rapidly more. In Ratheesh, the infection was ripping through, without warning or concern, laying waste his heart, kidneys and brain. Multiple organ failure ushered death to the doorstep as Ratheesh moved into Stage 6 of Baveno, and we stood numb—watching as he drowned in darkness that we could not see but he felt.

Inside the ICU, we tried to figure out what was hurting Ratheesh, who was now battling death. A potent and highly drug-resistant bacteria called *Enterobacter cloacae* was in his blood—a condition called bacteremia—which was associated with a high death rate during the same admission. Antibiotics were pumped in as the ICU doctors struggled to keep Ratheesh alive. But then, shockingly, but also with grave expectations, the medicines did their work. To everyone's relief, his blood pressure stabilized in a few days, and his brain and kidney functions improved. But the jaundice had worsened, and his liver failure progressed without hope.

An infection had hurt his liver functions previously.

Now, a second, stronger one was dragging it down.

Back inside the hospital room, everyone was terrified, including the doctors, as Ratheesh battled to survive another day. Another attack of infection and Ratheesh would be gone—leaving behind his daughter and a loving wife. There was no liver donation in sight, and February was soon approaching.

I started hearing my old friend inside my head. Death's call. *It was etched in stone. Ratheesh had to go*. I felt it linger near my bed at home. Near me when I slept. Hanging around when I was lost in thought. It followed me because I was keeping something it wanted.

But then we were not willing to let go. Not yet.

~

One day, during the hospital rounds review, Ratheesh's little daughter, who was all this while so silent, spoke. She was only seventeen.

The future looked bleak.

Because she and her mother would be the only ones in it.

Her graduation would not be the same.

Her wedding would be morose.

A void was forming, taking shape, and was unfillable.

The sudden loss of a family member, especially the father, was a shot through her heart. She wanted to donate her liver. Her blood group was a perfect match. She was willing to get herself voluntarily evaluated for fitness to donate a part of her liver. But there was a great challenge: she was a minor. At seventeen years of age, and as per the rule of the land and legal binding, she was not yet an adult and had to be exempt from organ donation. But she wanted to donate. It was her father's life that was at stake. There was only one way. Approach a court of law.

So, with the help of an empathetic lawyer, the teenage girl, who wanted to see her father make it out alive, filed a petition. In it, she prayed to the Kerala High Court to allow her to donate a part of her liver willingly and with a clear mind to her dying father, even if she was a minor. This was something that had never happened in the country before. During the initial proceeding, the high court set up a committee from their side to investigate the matter. However, the committee saw that Ratheesh was in Stage D of BCLC, and they believed that a liver transplant would not be a good option for him in terms of long-term benefits—as per the algorithm. They missed the strategic exception that we held closely and were chasing rabidly.

They refused the girl's plea. But she would not stop. We would not, either.

Another plea was made—this time explicitly asking for an expert committee of liver specialists and not generalists. The honourable High Court allowed a repeat review from a new commission, which ruled in her favour. The new committee said that the girl was fearless, and their duty was to give her the chance to donate a part of her liver—because for her, it was worth everything. January was coming to an end, and the Kerala High Court did something never done before in India. 'Kerala Court Allows Minor to Donate Portion of Liver to Ailing Father,' read the news headlines in all major media.

Devi, the young girl, was taken up for a transplant surgery workup. However, something unexpected happened, dashing all hopes. Her liver was fatty. It had more than 20 per cent fat, and this had to come below 10 per cent for the surgeons to perform a safe surgery so that the harvested liver would work inside the patient, and the part that was left inside the young girl would be healthy enough to regenerate into a whole liver to help her body recover.

She had a month to do it.

If she did not lose weight and her fatty liver did not improve, then it was a devastating game over. Devi would have to attend her father's funeral within a month. Death would win, and love would lose. I spoke to her in my outpatient department. The nutritional science of weight loss was an art.

One can lose weight healthily and quickly through science and motivation, and I gave her advice on how to go about it. Portion control, caloric deficit and aerobic exercise, all wrapped in sustained dedication, were vital to weight loss.

She had to focus on only one person: her father.

'I want him to live,' she kept telling me, sometimes with teary eyes, sometimes lost elsewhere—maybe in her early childhood, maybe inside the photos kept at home. After a month of great motivation, an intense gym-based exercise regimen, a low-calorie diet and sacrificing everything sweet, Devi lost weight and came in for a re-evaluation. Her liver fat had dropped to below 10 per cent, and I signed the donor clearance. She was through, and the transplant surgery team took over the patient and the donor at the end of February. At seventeen years of age, Devi became the youngest liver donor and the first minor to donate a part of the liver in the country to an adult—for her father and to keep the family whole. Reviews at my outpatient department followed until the day of the transplant. In Ratheesh, we kept the dreadful Baveno Stage 6 at bay with great difficulty and an equal measure of dread.

Finally, the day came. Ratheesh's bad liver, with the gnawing tumour on it, went out.

Devi's young liver went smoothly into her father, giving him a new life.

Through the life he gave her, a part of it was given back to him, unconditionally.

Two weeks after the surgery, both the donor and the recipient went home, beating all odds. They went back to how it was before the nightmare, sharing an organ that was now regenerating at rapid speed to keep both their bodies alive.

There were ten days left in the month of February.

But no one cared.

We were not frightened anymore.

We did not let fear consume us.

When a child's love grew stronger than the foe it was to meet at the end, as doctors, we strove to deliver that promise at exhausting speeds—through the power of untiring medical science and human compassion.

A few days later, as I walked into my outpatient department and sat down to open the list of new patients I had to see that day, a website link popped up in my WhatsApp inbox from an unknown number.

I clicked on the link and looked at the headline. It was: 'How a 17-year-old Girl Donated her Liver to Save Dying Father.' It was published by *The Week* magazine on 4 June 2023.

I spent a few seconds reading the headline, closed the page and sat on my chair, lost in bittersweet thought, ending it with a smile.

I then proceeded to call my first patient.

I did not read the contents of that webpage.

Because I knew what it was all about.

I had lived it.

As Mother Teresa said, 'A life not lived for others is not a life.'

Don't Speak

'There is a referred case for you,' the emergency physician told me.

'How bad is it?' I asked him.

'Pretty bad,' came the pat reply.

'But nothing a good clinical history can't crack, eh?' I told him rather confidently.

'That seems to be the problem,' he shot back, 'the patient cannot speak. He is on the ventilator.'

At the previous hospital that he was admitted to, Navin, a forty-eight-year-old schoolteacher, did not give doctors time to figure out what was going wrong. He had presented to them with fatigue for one week, lacked interest in food and then, one fine day, become wholly disoriented and landed on the mechanical ventilator the very next day. Before he became disoriented, he had multiple episodes of vomiting, so much so that his family members saw death pouring out of him as he purged his insides. A collapse followed, and then severe dehydration; his skin felt like paper, and his blood pressure was unrecordable. After rushing in 2 litres of intravenous fluid, he was taken to the nearest hospital, where he was tubed (to protect his airways) and put on the mechanical ventilator. One, for the doctors to ensure that he remained stable and his organs were protected; and two, to buy them time to figure out what was happening inside Navin. This was a crisis. A healthy man had collapsed and was now fighting for life. And the worst part was that whatever was killing him was doing it rapidly.

The blood pressure was not picking up even after fluid had been pushed into his veins. Navin was in shock—a critical condition brought on by the sudden drop in blood flow through the body that may be a result of significant trauma, heatstroke, massive blood loss, severe allergy, overwhelming infection, poisoning or high-degree burns and other rare causes. There are mainly four types of shock: distributive, in which blood vessels are stunned due to an overwhelming cause; hypovolemic, due to blood or body fluid loss; cardiogenic, which is due to diseases of the heart; and obstructive, due to causes that reduce heart pump output, such as severe lung disease.

Doctors were quick to evaluate Navin for all causes of shock. The most common reason for shock is generally considered to be that which affects the whole body and blood vessels—due to overwhelming infection presenting in its worst form, called sepsis, which also results in multiple organ failure. Tests were done to identify the source of Navin's infection, and chest and abdomen imaging were performed immediately. Sepsis was reversible and could be cured—but only if they found the site or source of infection and identified the infecting organism. In time.

When the blood pressure was not picking up with large boluses of fluids, the doctors started medications to help maintain Navin's circulation, which also helped his heart beat. They initiated him on drugs called vasopressors and inotropes. Vasopressors are a powerful class of drugs that induce blood vessel constriction, and in the process, elevate body pressure. They differ from inotropes. The latter increase heart-pumping capacity. Many drugs have both vasopressor and inotropic action on the body.

Meanwhile, the extensive workup to identify a site or source of infection proved futile. Broad-spectrum antibiotics were started, considering a hidden and unrevealed site of infection. But even with the antibiotics, fluid therapy and drugs for blood pressure, Navin was not improving as expected. The doctors were now in a fix, as the rest of the blood reports started coming in—adding chaos to the already ongoing confusion. The ultrasound scan of the liver showed that it was coarse, with slightly irregular margins—features that were suggestive of chronic liver damage—and the sodium level in the blood was extremely low. Shock in a chronic liver disease patient with very low sodium (hyponatremia) was quite the critical situation. The physicians panicked because they lacked the expertise to manage Navin. And so, all hope intact, he was referred to us in a desperate attempt for a quick diagnosis.

First, we had to find the foe that was killing Navin, hiding in plain sight. Was liver disease the reason for all that was happening to Navin? We kept going through his medical history.

There had been warning shots. Navin was a teetotaller but had diabetes, which was well-controlled on medications. He did not have any additional risk factors for chronic liver disease. But we had to make sure. A liver biopsy was the gold standard for diagnosing chronic liver disease and cirrhosis. But Navin was too entrenched in a critical condition for us to be that adventurous. So we did something special—a non-invasive method that could help us rule out chronic liver damage. A simple imaging test, known as a shear-wave scan. It is an ultrasound technique that measures liver stiffness, helping us identify those with advanced chronic liver disease. The higher the stiffness, the higher the chances of the liver being chronically damaged. The low sodium is also a possible feature of advanced cirrhosis. However, this is rarely seen in the early stages of chronic liver disease. We noticed that Navin's liver stiffness was 5.4 kPa, meaning he did not have any underlying chronic liver damage. This added to our already increasing woes. What was causing the sodium to dip so low in this man?

My team was relatively quick to dismiss most causes of shock. There were no obstructions to heart-pumping or lung diseases, and heart and brain scans were normal. There were no identifiable or hidden causes for bleeding, and we found no identifiable source(s) of infection we could treat, which was both striking and worrying. We were left with something that was causing distributive shock in Navin, and the only clue we had to its reason was the low sodium. This became our focus. The approach to low sodium is one of the most challenging clinical scenarios in medical practice, making even the most experienced physician sweat blood and tears. Because low sodium could be tied to many diseases and many organ systems, this was one clinical event that forced everyone to remember everything from their medical training days.

But as physicians, we have help and hope and that is where the beauty of applied clinical algorithms in diagnosing disease lies. So we sat down and applied the algorithm to analyse the reason for the low sodium in Navin. First, we had to identify the low sodium type concerning the patient's clinically relevant fluid (volume) status. Here, Navin was severely dehydrated—so it was called hypo-osmotic, or low sodium associated with low fluid volume. Next, we checked the urine osmolality (the concentration of all chemical particles found in the fluid), and it was high, meaning sodium was being wasted into the urine and thus its level in the body was getting low. This can happen with kidney disease or failure, a resolving kidney failure due to the use of a group of drugs called thiazides, obstruction to urine flow at the various structural levels in the urine-genital system and in very low thyroid-functioning states. But Navin's blood work was clean for all of these.

Blood never lies. We were now left with the last few causes that the algorithm guided us towards. The first was a disorder called the syndrome of inappropriate antidiuretic hormone secretion (SIADH). In this condition, the body makes too much of a chemical called the antidiuretic hormone (ADH). This hormone helps kidneys control the amount of water our bodies lose through urine. The SIADH causes the body to retain too much water. This means that the fluid and volume status of the body would be high, and urine output would be low. But in Navin's case, volume status was low and urine output was normal. To our disbelief, SIADH was not a possibility. The next possibility was a condition called 'cerebral salt wasting', in which a brain infection or trauma or a stroke event results in sodium wastage in the urine, but in the presence of a high urine volume. In Navin's case, the urine volume was normal, and there was no brain event preceding the current clinical situation. So we focused on another disorder the algorithm led us to: mineralocorticoid deficiency. Mineralocorticoids are hormones that maintain the body's balance of sodium and potassium salts, keeping blood pressure normal. However, one more critical finding in mineralocorticoid hormone deficiency and its association with low sodium had to be the high potassium. So we looked at the potassium trends in Navin, from his first admission to the current one.

The initial potassium was low and did not fit in with what we were expecting.

'But the patient was vomiting heavily at the time,' my colleague told me.

And he was right.

Excessive vomiting resulted in potassium loss, which meant that the initial low potassium that Navin's blood work showed may not have been true. So blood *did* lie. We ran through subsequent reports and found that potassium was normal when the patient was shifted to us. This also did not make sense because Navin received no potassium correction or potassium-rich fluids during his move. We repeatedly looked at Navin's potassium levels at our centre, and lo and behold, it returned high. The serum potassium level in him was 6.8 mmol/L, higher than the 5.5 mmol/L limit. At our centre, Navin's potassium levels always remained high, but the initial vomiting, the fluid therapy, the drugs and the antibiotics had all masked an accurate investigational picture.

Now we had a diagnosis.

And we called it the Addisonian crisis.

~

The adrenals are two small glands located just above the kidneys, as described by Eustachius in 1714. Adrenal glands secrete mineralocorticoid hormones. In slow progressive destruction of adrenals, patients develop Addison's disease due to deficiency of these hormones. In 1855, Dr Thomas Addison described this condition, currently known by his name. In the majority affected, Addison's disease is usually slow to progress, diagnosed late and presented variably (including behavioural changes). Many patients are misdiagnosed as 'psychiatric' or 'depressed', and put on pills to help improve mental health, until someone figures out it is the adrenal glands and not the brain that is the real problem. However, if the damage to the adrenal glands occurs rapidly, it is called the Addisonian crisis. Both the adrenal gland functions could be destroyed rapidly due to an event such as a bleed or an infection, dampening their activity very quickly, leading to a medical crisis. If not identified on time, the crisis can lead to coma and death.

We had this knowledge now. Navin was possibly in a severe Addisonian crisis. He was dying fast on that ventilator, and we did not know what was causing it. To add to the complexity of the condition, and because medical science treats the body as a whole to find the root cause of diseases (unlike other supposed medical-care practices), we knew that another master gland—called the pituitary gland—in the brain controlled the adrenal glands. If the pituitary function was low, this would also lead to low adrenal function, known as secondary adrenal insufficiency.

However, the pituitary gland function can be normal and the adrenal glands could still be low-functioning, in a condition called primary adrenal insufficiency (caused by a disease of the adrenal glands themselves and not due to a disease outside of it). To identify this, there was another medical algorithm we had to apply. We saw that, in Navin, the hormone adrenocorticotropic (ACTH) from the pituitary was relatively high, and another hormone called cortisol (secreted by the adrenal gland) was low—which meant that the disease was primarily that of the adrenal glands. If it were due to the pituitary gland, the ACTH levels would have been low too. Armed with this newfound information, we started treating Navin for Addisonian crisis—to salvage his life. This meant lots of fluids, high doses of steroids that the adrenal gland was supposed to secrete but was not able to, maintenance of glucose levels in the body and most importantly, maintaining the blood pressure—all the while hunting for the cause of the adrenal gland failure.

What was causing Navin's adrenal gland damage? The most typical cause in India is chronic infection with the bacteria that causes tuberculosis. Yes, this bacteria can affect the adrenal glands and reduce their functioning, leading to Addison's disease or crisis. But a complete workup for infections was negative in Navin multiple times. A CT scan of the abdomen at the outside hospital was essentially normal. But something was missing.

There had to be something hitting Navin's adrenal glands.

We had a dictum. A rule of sorts in our department of diagnostics: Never feel bad repeating an investigation if it might open new doors, and never bank on another physician's conclusion if the diagnosis was still unclear, even if they were senior and experienced.

And so, we decided to repeat the CT imaging at our centre. Meanwhile, Navin was fighting on the ventilator. He was on multiple drugs to maintain his blood pressure. Even with all that assault on his body, his kidneys were doing well and his lung functions were stable.

But for how long?

The longer he spent time on the ventilator, the higher the risk of infections—it was only a matter of time before Navin's lungs would be hit by a multi-drug-resistant bug from the hospital. Once that happened, we would have to fight an unknown bug and a known sinister one, making the fight so much worse. With Navin on multiple organ support and the mechanical ventilator, an expert team of doctors shifted him for a CT scan of the abdomen and waited for the radiologist to give us a provisional report.

'The abdominal scan looks essentially normal,' my radiologist told me over the phone as I slumped back on my chair inside my office, completely lost. I felt useless.

All my life, I have studied medicine. I did not know anything more. I had to teach myself to sleep every day. Watching a movie or going out with friends was a luxury; my patients were always on my mind every single time. The only time dopamine rewarded me, my serotonin levels made me happy and my adrenaline gave me a thrill was when I diagnosed a patient, got him well and sent him home to a family that was waiting for him. The medical system ensured that my feelings remained in this vicious cycle of bittersweetness. And when that did not happen, as a doctor, I started to feel like I was not in my playground anymore and wanted out. The burnout was honest and brutal. I was getting deep into it, was getting old quicker than my body was showing.

My life made sense, but then it did not.

My phone rang. It was my radiologist again. 'But if you want me to make some additional comments and take a hard and close look at the adrenals, I would say they're not normal.'

I sat up and asked him, 'What do you mean not normal?'

'I mean,' he said, 'they look bulky.'

'Do you think we should needle it?' I asked him, wondering if he would be okay with going for a biopsy from the adrenals to see what was happening inside.

'What else you got to get going on?' he told me. 'Your tests pointed towards the adrenals, so adrenals are where you need to look deeper.'

'Would you do a biopsy from the adrenals for me?' I asked curiously.

'Yes, of course,' he complied. A moment of silence, and then: 'Like right now?'

'Yes.'

'But I need consent.'

'Leave that to me.'

I rushed out of the room to find Navin's family and discuss their next steps. 'Sir,' the son told me, 'We have been here almost a week. Appa has been the same.'

I sheepishly and embarrassedly told them, 'I am sorry, but the diagnosis was not simple—'

The son interrupted, 'No, what I meant was that he is still alive! He is still on the ventilator and on many supports, but he is with us. The doctors at the other hospital said he would not last twenty-four hours and would die of multiple organ failure. But your team has dragged his life with everything you got, taking him to almost a week.' His eyes filled with tears. 'For us, this is a miracle. Tell me, where do I sign?'

I looked at him and learnt a lesson. Sometimes, some illnesses are unbeatable. Some cannot be diagnosed on time. Patients die. But the process matters. I spoke to the family like a human—not like a doctor or a healer who sat high on a pedestal. I told them my worries. My concerns. My process. The algorithm. I had planned it, but I was still unsure and insecure about how the patient would respond. We were all on the same page. And this was what mattered. Not winning. Not losing. If the doctor's fight is patient-centric, a journey alongside the patient's family and not just a robotic routine process, then it is a battle already won, come what may. If the patient dies, then they know that I, too, die a little inside.

Our grief was one.

Communication was key.

Before he was shifted to the ICU, Navin's adrenal gland biopsy was completed under the CT scan guidance.

Finally, we saw it under the microscope in the pathology department. We saw what was killing Navin. We knew how to kill it back, but we had to find out how he had got it in the first place. So we returned to his family and asked about recent changes in Navin's life.

Navin had returned from the Middle East and started working as a teacher for his local village school. Nine months before his current ordeal, he had bought some excavated land and started small-scale cultivation activities near his village. He wanted to make a small sit-down area where students could take special classes. The area was dusty and thickly surrounded by trees, well known for flocking birds and bats. Navin cleared and cleaned off large sections dirtied by bird and bat excreta to arrange a teaching set-up and cultivate the land around it. He already had diabetes, and in the process, he was at risk for what Samuel Taylor Darling identified in 1905.

Samuel Taylor Darling was an American pathologist and bacteriologist. While working on parasites, he came across what he thought was the organism that caused malaria, but it was not as it seemed. The same organism he had found, we saw under our microscope too; one that can be inhaled and spread through infected bats and bird droppings. Under the microscope, we saw that Navin's adrenal gland was teeming with numerous tiny oval-shaped fungi with yeast forms and thin walls: *Histoplasma capsulatum.* It caused the disease known as Histoplasmosis, which is usually an affliction of the lung. It presents with acute pneumonia or can come in a disseminated form too, in which multiple organs (including the adrenal gland) can be affected. Histoplasmosis was also called Darling's disease or Caver's disease.

Pure adrenal gland presentation of Histoplasma was infrequent, and Addisonian crisis due to adrenal Histoplasma was an even rarer sight—one that had hit Navin without warning.

Now that we had found the cause, antifungal therapy was started. The beauty of treating infectious diseases was that the little critters melted away when we pushed anti-microbial drugs into the patient. It was a sight to watch. A marvel of medicine. Only in a matter of a few days, Navin's organ support started to come down and his blood pressure stabilized without the need for supportive medications. He was weaned off the ventilator, shifted out of the ICU and then transferred to a hospital room, where he spent twelve days under the watchful eyes of the ICU physicians.

Navin was discharged on long-term oral anti-fungal drugs after his rehabilitation in the hospital was complete.

~

A year later, during his final visit, I told him that he didn't need to come to my outpatient for any further follow-up, and that he was disease-free.

Before he left, he said, 'You are a liver disease specialist. I did not have liver disease. Why did you and the team take care of me?'

A momentary pause, and then I remembered.

My professor in medicine would be very upset about one single matter when it came to patient care.

Patients survive.

Patients die.

Doctors have little control over many things when it comes to practical clinical medicine. But they have full control when they know the diagnosis.

'You do not let a patient die without knowing what is killing them,' my wise professor had told me.

A diagnosis is half the battle won. A diagnosis gave closure to many, even if they eventually passed on. If they did not know, their family would know. A diagnosis gave them comfort because they would make peace with the fact that everything was done to win a life back.

'I could not let you die. Not without knowing and facing what was hurting you,' I told Navin.

'Can I visit you sometime, even if I am healthy?'

I asked him, 'Why? People usually hate coming to the hospital, especially healthy ones.'

He told me, 'Maybe to say hello. I do not know, but seeing you, this place, this room. I see light at the end of the tunnel. It is warming.'

As I smiled at him and nodded, I thought of algorithms.

Rebirth

My staff ushered in a man and his mother, cradling a fragile, small-framed five-year-old boy into my outpatient department.

I looked at my list and asked, 'Mr Ram?'

The staff told me that Mr Ram was next on the list, but this boy looked very sick and had been given priority. I looked at the boy. And then at the man and the older woman cradling the child. I felt shivers down my spine and knots developing inside my stomach.

And I knew what this was.

A race against my worst enemy.

Time.

The boy's name was Dheeraj, which, in Sanskrit, meant 'patience'.

But this was not a time to be patient because if we lost time, we lost the little patient.

~

Dheeraj was diagnosed with a dreadful liver condition called biliary atresia a few weeks after birth. It is a blockage in the tubes (ducts) that carry bile from the liver to the gall bladder. This congenital condition occurs when the bile ducts inside or outside the liver do not develop normally. The bile stagnates inside the liver, leading to progressive and severe inflammation and damage to the liver cells, which then causes scarring and rapid onset cirrhosis in children.

The most common reason for liver transplantation in children in the world is biliary atresia. The condition presents in the immediate period after birth and is indicated by persistent jaundice, clay-coloured stools and a large liver. The clay-coloured stools are entirely characteristic of this disease in newborns. Typically, the liver releases bile salts into the stool, giving it a standard brown colour. But when the bile production or flow is reduced (such as in biliary atresia), the release of bile salts into the intestines decreases, leading to a change in the colour of stool to that of a peculiar clay-white. Biliary atresia is fatal if left untreated, with a reported survival of less than 10 per cent at three years of age. The disease affects one in 8,000–18,000 live births worldwide. The whole idea of active treatment is to let the bile flow so that the liver cells do not get damaged by the stagnation and inflammation in the long term. This helps prevent a condition called chronic cholestatic liver disease, which can result in advanced cirrhosis and liver failure.

To get the bile going in Dheeraj, a surgery was performed called the Kasai procedure, named so after the Japanese paediatric surgeon Morio Kasai, who developed it in 1950. Dheeraj underwent the procedure when he was forty-two days old. Everything seemed fine until the infections arrived without warning. Cholangitis, or infection within the bile duct system, was a dreaded complication. When it occurred repeatedly, the expected benefits of the Kasai surgery failed. When the jaundice had not resolved even six months after the procedure, the doctors advised Dheeraj's parents to opt for a curative liver transplantation if the infections kept recurring and the organ started showing signs of failure. The family was distraught. They had spent a good amount of money on the Kasai procedure and hospitalization for the repeated infections, and now there was no way they could afford a liver transplant.

Every time they met the doctors during the child's follow-up visits, they would always talk about a liver transplant and nothing else.

They were tired of those words. Liver transplantation.

Desperate, they took the next best option.

One they thought was safe, natural and effective without side effects.

One that always came as a saviour when modern medicine and medical science failed.

The great hope that flowed through social media and by word of mouth. Relatives, neighbours and friends vouched for it, and even the government promoted it.

What could go wrong?

It was as old as time itself.

It thrived on anecdotes and personal experiences.

Ayurveda.

The Ayurvedic practitioner looked at the child and said, 'This is not biliary atresia but a disease arising from problems with Kamala and Pandu.'

In ancient and primitive Ayurvedic texts, these terms were used to describe a group of diseases that 'resembled' jaundice or presented with jaundice. There is no realistic cause for jaundice described within these texts, and such ancient practices in the modern world are based on appeal to antiquity and traditions, not scientific inquiry and reform.

Dheeraj underwent intense herbal treatments, massages and highly restrictive dietary therapies that were supposed to cure his congenital liver disease without the need for surgery. The boy was given a bunch of herbal supplements—of which some were labelled, others unlabelled—over a period of three long years for the 'Kamala' disease. He was put on a constrained dietary regimen, which triggered avoidant restrictive food intake disorder in his parents. They were systematically dragged into and suffered fearmongering about harmful foods and foods that were healing, a wholly unscientific nutritional practice. Animal-based proteins were restricted, a plant-based diet was initiated, and the nutritive value of consumed food was heavily curbed. Even with a failed Kasai surgery, children do well for a few years, as per the natural history of the disease, when a plateau phase occurs. Thereafter, the phase of progression kicks in. Once the disease progresses, with a background of malnutrition that serves as a ticking bomb for repeated infections, it snowballs into a rapid decline of health, which culminates in the death of the child.

When the family saw that after starting the Ayurvedic treatments, Dheeraj was seemingly 'stabilized', they lost all hope in modern scientific medical therapies—ignorant about the fact that the disease had plateaued as per its natural history and the child was ageing.

But he was not growing.

His bones became brittle.

His liver disease progressed more rapidly in the presence of long-term use of possibly toxic and untested herbal supplements. In three years, Dheeraj became highly malnourished, and his growth was stunted.

~

When I saw him in my outpatient room, he was slipping into a coma triggered by the liver failure, curled up within the comfort of his grandmother's arms. He was a five-year-old, but looked like and weighed as much as a one-year-old. He was very sick, and I knew that the failed Kasai and years of alternative medicine and witchcraft-like treatments, along with malnutrition, were killing his liver. We had no luxury of waiting for him to improve with only medical optimization. As the next best step, we rushed him into the paediatric ICU where—along with a team of excellent residents and doctors—the boy was quickly evaluated for every possible nutrient deficiency. On the side, we managed his brain failure triggered by the high ammonia, which had been precipitated by the liver failure. Infections were screened for and treated. The malnutrition became the most challenging part for us to handle, since we had to prevent a condition called 'refeeding syndrome' in Dheeraj. This condition results in potentially fatal shifts in the fluids and electrolytes (such as sodium, potassium and magnesium) in malnourished patients receiving proper nutritious food after a prolonged period of starvation. As the tiny body was not used to proper nutrition, adequate feeding can make it go haywire, sometimes leading to life-threatening events that can kill the child. We did it slow and steady, without hurting the child, who was supposedly recovering.

The most important part of our management was quenching our curiosity about knowing how soon Dheeraj would require a liver transplant. And what better way than to ask the liver itself? A liver biopsy was called for. But with the liver failure, there was no way we could go for a direct liver biopsy due to the high risk of life-threatening complications. As Dheeraj was so malnourished and protein deficient, the lack of clotting factors would trigger bleeding into his small liver. We found another way and called in the experts. Our group of interventional radiologists accessed Dheeraj's liver through a vein in the neck (transjugular method, as described in previous chapters) using a unique set of tools and techniques once the child was mildly sedated. A masterful biopsy was performed by the interventional physicians under extreme stress, sweat, blood and tears.

Once the liver-biopsy reports came in, we saw that the biliary atresia had progressed to cirrhosis, and the liver cells were extensively damaged due to stagnant bile along with the super-added herbal assault that the poor child's liver had been subjected to over the years. Two insults were happening at the same time within the liver, which had triggered a relentless liver failure.

This meant only one thing. The need for a liver transplantation to keep Dheeraj alive was the priority.

Living-related donor liver transplantation was the best option, since the chances of getting a cadaver liver during the pandemic were almost zero. So the family started to look for relatives who were willing to donate a part of their liver to save Dheeraj. The mother had just given birth to a baby girl, so she was ticked off the list. Dheeraj's father did not match because his blood group was different. Theirs was a small family, and all the helter-skelter activity was not giving them the hope of finding a liver donor among relatives. Without an immediate liver transplantation, a curative intent was impossible, which left us with one last option—best supportive care to improve the quality of the little life that was left, until the child died of natural causes due to advanced liver disease.

Unable to bear the devastating news, the silent old grandmother—who had been the child's pillar of strength—volunteered to be the liver donor. Her blood group was a match. But she was a frail elderly lady. We told her that even though it was a risk worth taking, it was still a significant risk to her life and the child. An older liver may not regenerate on time, killing the boy, and if the remnant liver would not regenerate adequately in the donor it would also kill her. The older woman had never been more confident about a decision in all her life. Seeing her courage, love and strength, our transplant team gathered the confidence to evaluate her. Miraculously, she passed all the stringent donor-screening criteria that ultimately made her the chosen liver donor for Dheeraj.

Meanwhile, Dheeraj was now fully stabilized after weeks of hardships from our medical team. His nutritional status had improved, and he had become more active. His brain failure subsided, and there was a glimmer in his near-dead eyes that I had witnessed on that first day. And here he was, ready to receive a part of his grandma's liver, with all the love that came with it.

~

A part of the gentlewoman's liver was carefully dissected out.

The ugly, deformed, nodule-peppered, green-stained, irregular liver from Dheeraj came out. Ever so gently, the transplant surgeons inserted a part of the donor's liver into Dheeraj, who was sleeping on, supported by a ventilator and watched over by expert anaesthetists who would make sure that he remained alive on the machine and woke up afterwards.

What is clinical medicine without humanity? Nothing more than the hollow, discarded bricks of an empty structure that becomes soulless and collapsing. Medicine, more than any other profession, transcends age, gender, caste, creed, race, religion, politics, and tradition and culture. It is a rare realm where action matters more than identity. The art of medicine thrives on clarity—on doing what needs to be done without distraction or bias.

A doctor who remains a lifelong student will always be a better practitioner. The moment a physician stops learning; the clarity of practice begins to blur. True meaning in medicine emerges when science is practised with rationalism and guided by empathy. Patients suffer, families despair and physicians burn out when compassion is absent. Yet when human connection is present, the family—the often-overlooked core pillar of patient care—becomes a powerful ally. Young or old, when people give in to the act of saving another, the practice of medicine becomes the thread that binds them together. Their decisions, shaped by trust in the doctor, can shift outcomes. But that trust only grows when a physician carries not just knowledge, but a deep love for humanity, even in the darkest moments. That love, more than anything, is what keeps medicine alive.

They stitched the little blood vessels, created a bile-drainage system and released clamps.

The tiny liver came alive as blood and bile flowed through it.

The fruit of labour from weeks of hard work from physicians.

Driven by intense expertise in interventional radiology.

Deep support from the liver pathology team.

Extreme dedication from the liver transplant surgeons.

Unending love from the family.

And an older woman's dream of seeing her little grandson survive and grow to become a healthy young man.

Little Dheeraj went home to hug his grandmother, carrying inside him a part of her for life.

As Emily Dickinson said, 'Unable are the loved to die, for love is immortality.'

A Million Kisses

'Hepatology case?' I asked the emergency physician on the other end of the call.

'Not sure, doc,' he replied. 'Severe pancreatitis, but something is off. I think your unit needs to look at it. The liver looks coarse, and there is fluid in the abdomen.'

We prepared ourselves for a confrontation so sinister that it left us breathless, gasping and clutching at the last straws to save life against an unspeakable disease.

We were oblivious to the shattering outcome that was coming at us, and the dread that it would bring us.

~

Jasmine had been a healthy thirty-nine-year-old mother of two children—a pretty ten-year-old girl and a handsome five-year-old boy. Her husband worked as an office staff for a large multinational company. Loss of appetite was her first symptom, followed by abdominal discomfort. These continued for over a month until she realized it was not something that would pass by.

An ultrasound scan of the abdomen was done at a nearby clinic, where she was brought in for initial evaluation, and it revealed a 'coarse-looking' fatty liver.

'It is just gas,' the elderly physician reassured her and prescribed a medication called omeprazole to reduce her discomfort. It did reduce her symptoms for a while but did not wholly abolish them. Then, unexpectedly, the discomfort morphed into severe pain, which was intense at times. It was all over her abdomen and back. Her husband took her back to the same physician, who prescribed her another medication, called diclofenac, a powerful painkiller. Again, it helped her. But only for a while.

Then, two days later, the pain was back again, but worse. Only this time, her face was puffed up and her lower limbs were swollen. She was taken to a bigger, better nearby hospital, where the doctors who saw her in the emergency department started initial evaluations without haste.

The blood work showed high white cell counts and raised C-reactive protein, a marker of inflammation. A repeat ultrasound scan revealed something new, something crucial. A bulky pancreas and related blood reports revealed very high amylase and lipase enzyme levels. The pancreas is an elongated, tapered organ located across the back of the belly, behind the stomach, and surrounded by other organs—including the small intestine, liver and spleen. The organ produces certain chemicals, primarily enzymes, in the proper quantities at the correct times to digest our food. These enzymes include trypsin and chymotrypsin to digest proteins, amylase for the digestion of carbohydrates, and lipase to break down fats. When the pancreas is inflamed and swollen, the blood levels of the enzymes increase drastically.

In Jasmine, the diagnosis was straightforward—acute pancreatitis, a condition in which the pancreas becomes inflamed (swollen) over a short period. But something far worse was happening. Her kidney functions were deteriorating rapidly. The blood marker of kidney function, called creatinine, was high.

But, thought the doctors, *it is far too early for an organ failure to happen in acute pancreatitis.* This was only the second day of severe pain and the pancreatitis was not so severe, as per investigations. She had consumed a painkiller that was well known to cause kidney injury, but that was just one suboptimal dose. It could not be the cause for such severe kidney damage, the doctors were sure. There was no fluid in the abdomen and only a bulky pancreas without any destructive changes. The patient was not looking critically unwell, and her heart and lung functions were well maintained—except for the high heart rate due to dehydration and the pain. Acute pancreatitis can present in two distinct stages: one called interstitial pancreatitis, which means there is just swelling of the pancreas; the second, known as necrotizing pancreatitis, suggests that the organ tissue is damaged and has been replaced by 'necrotic' or dead tissue. The latter stage was of great concern because it was severe, and patients typically progressed to other organ failures.

To identify a necrotic pancreas, a CT scan was required. Not just any CT scan, but a contrast-enhanced CT, in which a dye is injected to light up the non-necrotic areas from the necrotic ones. But because Jasmine had poor kidney function, a dye-injected contrast CT could not be performed since contrast dye use could worsen kidney functions. A plain CT scan of the abdomen was ordered, which showed a mild, bulky, swollen pancreas with minimal fluid around it—which was not suggestive of severe pancreatitis. The liver looked fatty, but did not feature chronic damage and shrinkage.

What stumped the doctors was that the early kidney injury did not fit in with the current acute pancreatitis picture. It should not have happened this early, and other causes for kidney injury were non-contributory on tests. Nonetheless, the doctors had what they wanted and decided to treat Jasmine as a case of severe pancreatitis based on a set of clinical criteria called the Revised Atlanta Classification. Treatment included aggressive fluid therapy, since severe dehydration and fluid sequestration in the body could lead to kidney injury. Acute pancreatitis and its sequelae can go on for close to six weeks. Most deaths happen within the first two weeks due to severe inflammation and associated organ failure. Early management is of great importance. But strangely,

Jasmine's kidneys simply didn't respond. Even with aggressive and well-reasoned fluid therapy, the expected recovery never happened. This was now a more significant challenge, and a repeat abdomen ultrasound was ordered again, considering the rapidly progressing disease evolution.

But the pancreas still looked the same: bulky and with very little fluid around it. Even though confused, the doctors decided to continue fluid-only management and rest the pancreas by not allowing the patient to take food orally. A feeding tube was inserted into the small bowels through her nose, and nutrient-rich feeds were given to Jasmine every few hours. Despite the aggressive course of treatment, the disease took another unexpected turn when complete kidney failure kicked in and Jasmine started to experience meagre urine output. Her kidneys were shutting down fast. To relieve the load on the kidneys and prevent the patient from going into complications associated with kidney failure—such as uremia (toxin build-up in blood) and high potassium and its related life-threatening consequences—a session of dialysis was performed. The patient stabilized and then was shifted to our hospital for further care.

~

'Hepatology case?' I asked the emergency physician on the other end of the call.

'Not sure, doc, but I think your unit needs to take a look at this.'

I looked at Jasmine lying on the green-sheeted bed inside the emergency room. The dialysis lines were going in and out of her neck veins. She was conscious but drowsy, and her heart rate was through the roof. Quite breathless, her state was proof that kidneys were severely dysfunctional. Her abdomen felt 'doughy', and her bowel sounds were sluggish and not frequently audible. She winced in pain when I lightly touched her abdomen.

'All classic signs of severe pancreatitis,' my colleague told me.

'This is not a hepatology case. Let us transfer her to gastroenterology and the ICU guys,' my other colleague chipped in.

But I was not ready to let go. Something was calling. Something that was left unspoken. Something unfinished. I had to be there. It was not my calling. But I made it mine.

'Let us keep her,' I told my colleagues. 'Something is off. I do not feel good about handing over her care. There is something waiting to be found.'

We reordered a plain CT scan of the abdomen, which showed the same findings the doctors at the previous hospital witnessed: a swollen pancreas with minimal fluid around it.

However, this did not fit with the clinical stage of organ failure.

What was happening? we all pondered. There were many causes for acute pancreatitis. We had ruled out almost every single one of them at the outset.

The most common was gall bladder stones that came out and blocked the pancreatic duct, causing enzyme build-up inside the pancreas and damaging its tissue. Then came alcohol use and infections. But all these had been explicitly ruled out.

Except one.

Cancer of the pancreas. Large tumours on the pancreas can block the pancreatic duct and obstruct the enzyme flow, resulting in acute pancreatitis. However, to confirm these details, we needed a contrast CT scan. After thirty-six hours and one more session of dialysis, Jasmine's abdomen started to distend like a balloon. She was too sick to be moved to the radiology department for a CT scan. I clinically examined her abdomen again. The repeat examination strangely suggested an 'increasing doughy feeling' of the abdomen. An ultrasound was performed, and this time something new and sinister entered the frame. The peritoneum (a membrane lining the cavity of the abdomen and covering the abdominal organs) and another structure called the omentum (the large, flat fatty-tissue layer nestling the surface of the organs) were also thickened.

'Oh, well, this can happen in severe pancreatitis as the disease progresses and when the inflammation spreads inside the abdomen,' said my colleague.

'But look, there is no fluid collection, and the pancreas still looks just swollen,' I countered.

There were no features to suggest why this was severe necrotizing pancreatitis, even though Jasmine's condition was clinically behaving like one. However, we had not done a contrast CT scan of the abdomen to check for necrosis. Both her kidneys were fried, and she was already on dialysis. Since the kidney support was ongoing, we could technically do the contrast-dye-injected CT scan. We needed to rule out pancreatic cancer too, even though ultrasound screening and blood work did not give vital clues. We walked around the waiting area and found Jasmine's husband and their children in tow on either side.

'Hello, sir,' I told him. 'We need to do a CT scan of the abdomen with contrast dye injection. Her kidneys are already bad, and since she is on dialysis, the dye could make it worse, but the dialysis will help. I am sorry that we have no options left to get to the bottom of what is hurting her.' I did not mince my words.

'We do not know what is hitting her this hard,' my colleague told him.

The husband looked up and asked, 'Will this help us find a cause?'

I said, 'Probably, but the cause could be something terrible, which we may not be able to treat.'

The husband, now a weary man, his eyes so tired, but his mind so sharp even in the face of an intense life-threatening challenge to his wife's health and to the mother of his kids, told me, 'Sir, I am not sure how this is going to end, but please, at least tell me what is killing my wife, so that I can make my kids understand that we all tried ... I tried.' He paused for a while.

'Please, give us closure,' he said, his eyes pleading.

At that moment, I remembered something.

The art of medicine was not about doing everything for the patient you were losing but also everything for the family—a chance to complete their story. That was why, even though this was not my case, I felt as if the universe had conspired to put me there. It had given me the responsibility and an opportunity to diagnose this woman and find ways to save her life for the sake of her children and that loving man who would miss her very much.

This would be their story. And I was here to complete it.

The contrast CT of the abdomen opened more questions than answers. It gave a death blow to the only possible diagnosis we had in mind. There was no cancer of the pancreas, and everything on that scan was precisely what was suggestive of pancreatitis on the previous scans. There was no necrosis and no progression to necrotizing pancreatitis. Just that same old swollen pancreas; swollen, thickened omentum and peritoneum layers; minimal fluid; and a few enlarged lymph nodes or abdominal glands—all features associated with severe pancreatitis. The patient was crashing. Her kidneys needed continuous dialysis support—through a process called CRRT, or continuous renal replacement therapy. A lot of money was being spent. And for nothing.

I felt like a loser. I felt bitter about my role. I was not helping Jasmine or her husband further than they were already helped. As her clinical status worsened, we had to put Jasmine on a ventilator to reduce her pain and improve her lung function. We were letting her hold on with so much organ support. Time was running out for us to get to a diagnosis, to a closure.

I did not meet her husband that evening during rounds. My colleagues did that for me. Even though I saw him sitting in the lobby with his children, looking over the central garden, I slipped out of the hospital through the back door inside the emergency room—exactly where I had seen and admitted Jasmine first—and drove home. I did not know what to tell him. I had nothing more to offer him, other than comforting words. But they would not mean anything to him. My words would hardly dent the grief he was trying to come to terms with.

Back home, I unwound, played with my children and discussed the weekend plans with my wife. But at the back of my mind, Jasmine's husband's words played in a loop. And their children's faces, like a slideshow, came and went. I did not know what to tell him the next day. His wife would only survive a few days longer, and I did not understand what was happening. He would go home with his children to bury their mother, who would turn into a memory, and her death would remain a mystery. I lay on my bed, trying to sleep and avoid the troubles my mind was cooking up. It was as if I had failed a whole family who came to me for help and care. They only wanted me to know what was killing her.

I could not even do that. Was I really a doctor?

My wife was asleep and my children were too. I had forgotten a time when I had slept so quickly and well. I closed my eyes and played everything in my mind—from the moment I first saw Jasmine on that bed inside the emergency room to the resignation and fathomless pain in her husband's eyes now.

As I lost my sleep, in that darkly lit room, my mind woke up.

What were the rare causes of pancreatitis that we were missing?

Did we miss anything reversible?

One by one.

And again and again.

In my head.

I tried to remember every book I had read throughout the years.

Autoimmune pancreatitis, IgG4 disease. Ruled out.

Genetic causes for pancreatitis. Ruled out.

Pancreatic or abdominal cancers. Ruled out.

The rare eosinophilic pancreatitis. Ruled out.

Drugs causing pancreatitis. No chance. The clinical history was clean.

Roundworms can go up the pancreatic duct, causing pancreatitis. But we would have seen them.

Diseases affecting blood vessels (called vasculitis disorders). None had been detected.

Just so tragic. Damn everything. Everything was negative.

Then I tried to remember everything that the contrast CT scan of the abdomen had showed, as well as my discussion with the radiologist.

And then two words—two words—made me feel strange.

Why did the radiologist say it? Why did he put it that way?

He had said, 'The omentum and peritoneum are disproportionately thickened.'

Disproportionately thickened.

Why?

And I could not sleep.

I wanted tomorrow to come. Right away. Sleep was now a formal burden.

I had bigger things to do.

There was this family. They were waiting for a diagnosis and closure.

In that thought, I drifted away, mumbling, into a sleep-like state.

~

I left early for the hospital the next day. In the ICU, I saw that the team was struggling to keep Jasmine alive.

'How long until we lose her?' I asked the chief medical officer.

'If she survives seventy-two hours, it will be a miracle,' he told me.

Seventy-two hours.

That was all I had.

All I needed.

I went to my radiologist and asked him, 'Why did you say "disproportionately thickened"?'

He looked at me and said, 'I do not know. I have seen a lot of acute pancreatitis cases. However, this one had findings within the pancreas with very minimal severity. Seems strange that the omentum and peritoneum are thickened so much.'

'Can you biopsy the omentum?' I asked him.

'Why?' he asked, 'How would that even help us? In the best circumstances, it may only show inflammation.'

'I don't know,' I told him. 'But I want it done. Can you do it?'

And he said, 'Yes, but you need to get the husband to consent for a high-risk biopsy on his dying wife.'

I nodded my assent.

He continued, 'And do not forget to mention you are doing it without knowing why you are doing it.' He looked me dead in the eye. 'But if he is willing, I'll get it done.'

I searched for Jasmine's husband and finally got hold of him near the ICU counselling room. I told him that I needed a biopsy done on Jasmine's omental region inside the abdomen. I told him I did not know why I was doing it, but that I had to do it.

He looked at me and said, 'Do you think it will help us get her better?'

I told him, 'No. She is going to die. She has maybe seventy-two hours left.'

He dropped his gaze to his feet.

'But I want to tell you why she died.'

He looked back at me.

The tears in his eyes reflected the light; he was holding them back from flowing down.

To show he was strong, for his children.

And my heart beat fast.

So fast that my palms and forehead sweat.

'Okay,' he said.

I rushed to call my radiologist.

On a mechanically ventilated patient with multiple organ failure, my radiologist performed a bedside omental biopsy and sent it for pathology review on behalf of a distraught father and his children. This was a diagnosis all of us were searching for, to bring them—and ourselves—closure.

I could not mess this up. If I did, I would carry this burden all my life.

Thirty-six hours after the biopsy, during my evening outpatient work, I got a call from the ICU that Jasmine had crashed on the ventilator. Her heart had stopped beating, and she was not responding. I rushed to the ICU and saw cardiac compressions being done on an unresponsive Jasmine. Multiple doses of adrenaline were injected—a last attempt at reviving the young woman.

I went out and talked to the husband.

He asked, 'Can my daughter see her?'

The children had not seen their mother since she was on the ventilator.

I asked him, 'Do you want this image of their mother to be the last one they will remember her by? It is your call. I can allow it.'

He cried in front of me. He was not going to hold back those tears anymore.

He asked the children to stay outside while he and I both went to his wife, who was now unresponsive.

The ICU physician was readying to declare her time of death.

The husband held his wife's hand and squeezed it hard, sobbing quietly.

That squeeze.

I will never forget it.

I felt all the love he had for her.

Acknowledgement.

Thankfulness.

Gratitude.

It felt like a million kisses in a single moment.

I let them be and stepped out of the ICU.

As I stepped out, I got a call from my pathologist. And I felt the closure first.

Closure that we did what we could and there was nothing more.

And closure that we had finally found it.

Jasmine's omental biopsy revealed healthy omental fatty tissue, which was deeply infiltrated by many cancer cells. These cells underwent further special staining to identify their origin. They showed some strange features—a unique marker called the leucocyte common antigen, cMyc, CD 30 and CD 43 were positive; while the cytokeratin 7 and 20 markers were negative—suggestive of a cancer known as anaplastic large B-cell lymphoma, a terrifying cancer of the lymphatic system. Primary lymphomas are uncommon pancreatic cancers. They constitute less than 2 per cent of cancers occurring outside lymph nodes. Primary pancreatic anaplastic large cell lymphomas are extremely rare, with less than ten cases reported worldwide. Even rarer was anaplastic large cell lymphomas involving the pancreas secondarily—this is what had led to acute pancreatitis in Jasmine.

Ours was the first case in the world.

The lymphoid cancer cells had infiltrated Jasmine's pancreas, damaging it and leading to pancreatitis. After the death certification formality was completed and I finalized the death summary, I called the husband to hand over the papers to him one final time.

At the handover time, I opened the paper cover, unfolded the document and showed him the diagnosis.

I told him how bad a disease it was.

And he asked me, 'If we had diagnosed it earlier, while she was in hospital, would things have been different?'

I said, 'No, we would still have lost her because the disease was made for us to fail.'

He walked away, towing his children on either side of him.

And my eyes welled up.

I was on the brink of tears.

But I did not cry.

I would wait to get back home and get under my shower first.

Before leaving, Jasmine's husband had taken my hands into his own.

He had squeezed them ever so tightly.

And I felt it.

Acknowledgement.

Thankfulness.

Gratitude.

Closure.

As Frank Herbert said, 'There is no real ending. It's just the place where you stop the story.'

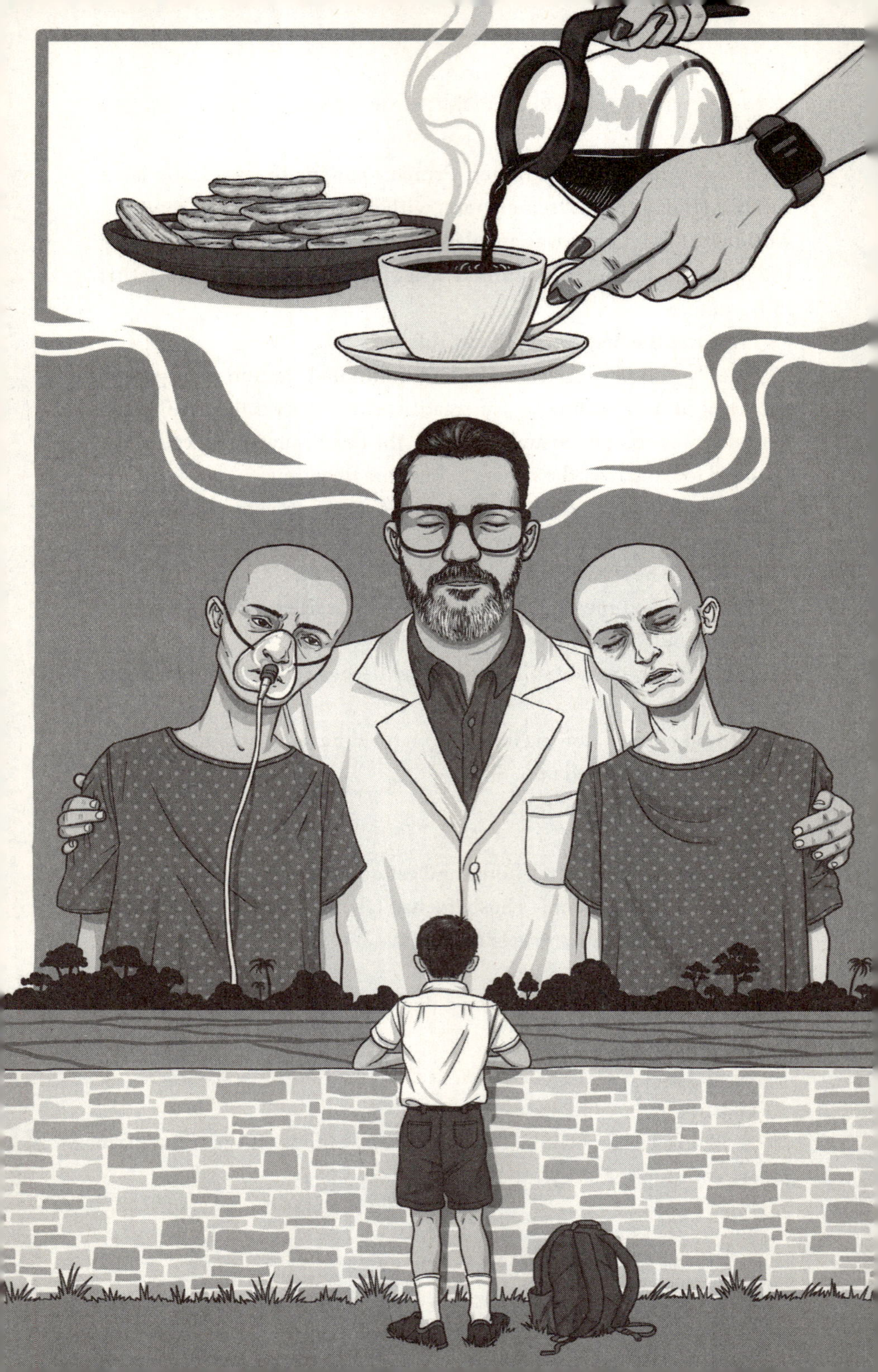

Epilogue
In Death, We Dream

Personal Heaven

DEATH. FROM THE TIME YOU ARE BORN, DEATH BECOMES your friend. When everyone else is moving away, Death is there for you. Watching and waiting, to gift that embrace that will not let go.

It was the June of 2023. A day like any other. I waited for a patient and his family to exit my outpatient room for the next in line to come in. Halfway through their exit, a middle-aged man ushered in a young girl across the doorway. She was nineteen years old. She was not jaundiced or lethargic. Even before he sat down for me to ask him details, teary-eyed, the man, her father, told me only one thing.

'She was advised to undergo a liver transplant to prolong her life. We were poor, and you helped us avoid it. Next week, she is going to join college. We wanted to see you before that. Thank you.'

I looked at Saikrishna. The young girl had been fourteen when I had diagnosed her after one of the most nerve-wracking and stressful weeks of clinical medicine practice in my career yet. As discussed earlier, when I first saw her, the class topper struggled to remember things. She was in the early stages of brain failure, with jaundice and struggling to get a life-saving liver transplant. Her studies were affected. A good student, she barely caught up with class assignments. Unintentional alcohol use from the Ayurvedic herbal formulations and chronic exposure to arsenic from the multiple herbal drugs had ravaged her mind and body. Her menstrual periods were irregular, and for months at a stretch, she did not have them. Her hair fall was intense, her face pigmented and hollow, and her eyes were visibly yellow for months. Now nineteen years old, she had come for her follow-up review with her father.

Nineteen years old.

Now, as she sat before me, she looked healthy and had put on weight, her skin pigmentation had resolved entirely, her hair was voluminous and shiny, and there was a sparkle in her eyes. Her menstrual cycles were regular, and she had never felt healthier in her life. Her father had a complete set of white hair and moustache. He looked at me and told me that I had grown old. I had aged almost six years. But I looked as if I had aged more than ten. The love, the regrets and the bittersweet regenerations—they were all peers on my playground. I sat before Saikrishna and her father with a thick salt-and-pepper beard and greying sideburns. I joked that her case added ten years to my life within the few weeks she was with me. Her father told me she had passed her twelfth grade with excellent marks and an A-plus distinction.

In a bittersweet moment, I was lost in thought and remembered what the same person had told me years ago: *She has been advised to undergo a liver transplant to prolong her life. We are poor. Can you please help us avoid it?*

She was starting a bachelor's degree in clinical psychology and was going to stay at a new hostel, making new friends and living a new life, away from her parents. Earlier, her father had searched exhaustively to find someone who would liberate him from all that darkness that shrouded him, and all the nightmares of loss that had engulfed his sleep. He had come to me after a great many ordeals at multiple hospitals, where every specialist had advised a liver transplant—the only way to save his daughter. All of them had told him that she would die in six months without a liver transplant.

That was nearly six years ago.

I asked her, 'Why clinical psychology?'

She told me, 'I do not know what treatments you gave me that helped me and saved my father from misery at the time. But you always listened to my father and mother and spoke to me with a smile. And you never showed us your worry even though you were worried. I want to listen to people and speak to them, to heal them. Like you did with me.'

I bade Saikrishna and her family goodbye. They remain in my heart.

There is no greater happiness than seeing your patient give back with love. Suppose there is an afterlife. Given a choice—even with all those hardships and the premature risk of dying from stress, poor life quality and loss of youth—I would still choose the life of a doctor, practising clinical medicine in the blink of an eye and the beat of a heart.

This is the life I chose to live.

Requiem for a Dream

I am at the beach today. It is a warm day. I am away from the hospital. My mind is clear, but my heart is heavy from the many scars that I embraced over the week. Some wounds hurt, and some are sweet, like a longing that refuses to let go—my patients who died, the ones waiting in the ICU to die and the ones who will be thrust into my care over the coming days. I am sitting on a soft beach towel that crumbles under me from time to time. My children are making shapes in the sand. My wife is looking at me from a distance. Her face is engraved into my mind.

A moment.

My children call out to me.

~

I remember now. It was November. The year was 2022. It was the festival of lights. Diwali. I was driving home late after work. It was a dark evening. The streetlight was not fully on. The roads were empty. I was cruising. My mind was on the road. But also, inside my ICU.

My patients.

Their families.

Children with liver disease.

Mothers on the ventilator.

Husbands hooked to dialysis machines.

Fathers readying to say goodbye.

Families torn because alcohol won.

Sons waiting by the ICU door.

Daughters crying because they were left to walk down the aisle alone.

My mind was not truly on the road.

I was inside my ICU.

My body was inside my car.

And that crash.

People say that your life flashes in seconds in the moment of death. As my car crashed head-on into the back of a large trailer truck parked on the side of the road, invisible to my vision because the streetlights were out, my life did not flash in front of me. But time seemed to slow down. I saw my phone swish past in slow motion over my shoulder, and the car deodorant bottle break into a thousand pieces. I saw the airbags deploy slowly around me, yearning to bag me in white. And then a sudden and forced stop, and the crash came to a halt. Everything was reduced to cinders.

But I was alive. Dazed and confused, I opened my car door and sat at the curb side while many people—and I do not know where they all suddenly came from; I swear the roads were empty except for that truck I did not see—started looking inside my totalled car for the remains of my body.

But I kept telling them I was the one inside and that I was not dead.

Not yet.

In that moment of death, I did not see my fears.

I saw my home. I saw people in it.

I saw everything go slowly.

It was as if the universe was telling me to slow down and see.

Open your eyes, see.

And I did.

You will remember the small things that mattered. Small things that you took for granted when the person was alive. The remembrance will turn into grief. The grief will grow. It will keep growing until it overwhelms you. You will cry your heart out because the tears are the only way you are allowed to channel regret. You will think that all those tears will help you see meaning; help you remember everything good. But the tears are a lie. They reinforce your loneliness, and time will not heal it. Like an unfair jury, time will give you new memories to replace your older, meaningful ones. You will never heal. You will forget the good things that once were. At one point, the good things cease and spark only when triggered. You will move on. Until the day you die. At the time of death, you will see them again. Only the best things. You will remember. Time and the universe that mocked you before, to give you closure, will make you see all the love that was, every little good thing, because that is the last thing you want to see.

I am at the beach.

My children are making shapes in the sand.

My wife is looking at me from a distance. Her face is engraved into my mind.

A moment.

My children call out to me. I am half-asleep, but my mind is with them.

My eldest daughter, Alanna, calls out to me, 'Papa, are you awake?'

~

I am a hepatologist.

Arguably, I care for the sickest group of patients in medical practice: end-stage liver disease.

I see death almost every day in my ICU.

Some are natural deaths resulting from multiple organ failure triggered by a failing liver.

Some are decided.

The family decided to pull the plug. They decided it was time to let go.

Every time I see my patient's heart rate drop, the blood pressure fall and the electrocardiogram go flat, I wonder, *What goes on inside a dying brain?*

Is it a small black hole that gets bigger and bigger and then engulfs the reducing field of light in absolute darkness as the heart shuts down, taking the brain away with it?

Or is it all light at the end of the tunnel and then darkness once the destination has been reached?

~

A group of doctors did something strange. Something unimaginable.

And it led to them witnessing something melancholic but beautiful.

They went inside an ICU and saw that four patients were unconscious. They were not clinically dead yet. And they weren't brain-dead. They were comatose. They were kept alive by a machine that pumped oxygen into their lungs. Three had brain injury due to cardiac arrest and lack of oxygen. One patient had haemorrhaged into his brain. All had been unresponsive for a very long time, and sadly, the families had decided to pull the plug on them.

To let them go away peacefully.

But before they did that, their loving families did something bittersweet. They signed a document that was made by the group of doctors, allowing them to study their beloveds' dying brain. Dr Jimo Borjigin of the Department of Molecular and Integrative Physiology, University of Michigan School of Medicine at Ann Arbor, led the group. The doctors fitted machines on the chest and head to study the heart and brain of the dying patients. Once all the machines were in place, they withdrew life support by removing the breathing tubes. Immediately after the tubes were removed, the dying patients' brain activity did not show anything different, nothing significant. But as their brains got closer to death, about 300 seconds before death, there was a sudden power surge. It occurred in the brain regions associated with conscious experience. As if the dying were suddenly yearning to live. Make no mistake, these were not 'some bursts' of electrical activity that happened when the brain cells withered away without oxygen.

This was a special kind of activity.

These power surges increased connectivity in a region in the brain called the posterior cortical 'hot zone'—an area crucial for conscious perception. When it came to the moments just before death, the brain cells were having a cross talk, not fading away into oblivion. The brain cells were passing final messages to each other within regions of the brain, while the physical body lay limp and motionless.

What the doctors had witnessed was bittersweet—because the final electrical pattern of the surges that the dying brains were showing were similar to those seen in dreaming humans.

All the patients in the study died.

But before they died, they taught us something.

That even in death, our minds are resilient.

That we clutch at only everything that was good.

What were they dreaming of?

A husband about his loving wife?

A mother her children?

Children, their parents?

Or maybe a scene from a movie that changed them? Or a song?

Or a pet who loved them unconditionally?

We will never know.

But know this: even in death, the mind conquers—with dreams and love, not nightmares and hate.

Remember, nothing perfect lasts forever except in our memories.

Make good memories while you are living so that you can relive them in death.

Hug your family.

Take your children for an ice cream.

Walk your dog into the sunset.

Sit on the beach.

Listen to the waves.

Hold your family close.

Conquer everything that has hurt you.

I think my children would have wanted me to play more with them.

But somewhere during the journey, I lost the child inside me.

I think clinical medicine did that to me.

Have you ever thought about what you will see, like a beautiful dream, right before the moment you die?

I know what I will see.

If you are reading this long after I am gone, you will know it too.

We will know what I saw.

Empty ventilators.

The ICU beeps, the blood and fluid lines.

Me stepping into a shower.

The flowing water on the floor tiles and my tears, indiscernible.

Kissing a Dalmatian's long face.

My wife's slender, petite, soft, nimble hands.

My children, all three, so young, and me not there.

That hot pot of coffee.

Freshly fried banana fritters.

My quaint little childhood town.

That school uniform. Navy-blue shorts and sky-blue checkered half-sleeve shirt.

Me in third grade.

That cute girl with big eyes who always gave me two Melody® candies for her birthday, when everyone else got one.

That petite girl, so fair, hiding the perfect set of teeth behind those thin pink lips.

Me making up lame jokes to see her smile.

That smile on her face.

That I lost them, except in my memories.

I am home.

Still in my school uniform, running towards a wall.

An old brick wall, just the perfect height.

Overlooking a rice field surrounded by water.

In the glistening water below, little fish with silver spots on their heads.

The breeze blowing gently through my short hair.

The drops of sweat on my forehead going cold.

That smile on my face.

Postface
Compromise

THIS BOOK WOULD NOT HAVE SEEN THE LIGHT OF DAY HAD IT not been for something terrifically important. As a physician and a subspecialist, arguably dealing with the sickest group of patients in medicine, it was an outlandishly difficult task for me to complete this assignment. Exhaustingly unnerving were the days, weeks and months that eventually culminated in the submission of the first draft of the manuscript. People asked me on Twitter about my secret plan that gave me time to watch movies; game on my desktop; and see, diagnose, treat and care for large, sick groups of patients every day. In between all that crushing post-work fatigue, I also found the time to agree to a book contract and then see it to completion.

The secret is called compromise.

I made many over the years.

These decisions did not happen one fine day, but slowly—they grew on me as I found clarity in confusion. I stopped seeing more than thirty patients in a day in my outpatient practice. I got out of the notion that a 'busy doctor' was a 'great doctor'. That people flock towards the busiest doctor because numbers are equivalent to expertise is a great myth in healthcare. The best doctors have time for their patients. Doctors are not shopkeepers who sell items or cashiers who account for products. It is a job, yes, I agree, but it is also about being dutiful. The time spent in asking all about the disease and its symptoms and checking for signs of the illness are not the most important part of clinical medicine practice. But spending time to *know the person* who harbours the disease is important. I stopped catering to 'hospital work things' after 5 p.m. until the next outpatient day, except when a liver transplant patient required additional attention. When I was home, I did not bring the hospital and patients with me into my family. I used to do that, but now I do not. It has helped me to love myself. Find time for myself. Many doctors forget who they really are because the work swallows them whole. They exist as a shell of their former selves, carrying within them work and its meandering remnants that never let go.

In my hospital practice, I focused more on admitting and caring for salvageable critically ill patients and stopped wasting the time and money of patients who were unlikely to make it. All they needed was comfort, not medicines. It changed the way I practised clinical medicine. I started using palliative care services for streamlining continued care of end-stage liver disease patients, since their recurring management, repeated admissions and exhaustive discussions with non-family members needed huge investments in the context of time and dedication.

Repeated discussions, especially when it came to death counselling, were burning me out. I found my limits—emotionally, mentally and physically. I stopped meeting pharmaceutical agents and pharma company representatives, as I found that reading a few hours every week on clinical updates was a far superior practice, which benefitted my patients more than me listening to medical representatives trying to sell their product based on their flimsy understanding of medical science. I understood that my clinical practice and experience did not suffer if this evening 'ritual' was discontinued.

I started trusting my colleagues and my team of doctors in making critical decisions for my patients. I stopped putting my fingers in all pies. From a professional standpoint, I stopped believing in the aspect of 'publish or perish in academic life'. I used to publish scientific papers very frequently, so much that a large part of my clinical research life was spent at home filling in Excel® sheets and analysing data, sacrificing the time I had for my children or that cup of coffee with my wife. I later understood that this was cruel. Not just on me, but on my family. I found myself moving away from this need of validation from academia and peers in medicine. I changed my routine and looked at publishing an academic study when I felt there was an important clinical research outcome that needed to be shared. I stopped publishing papers for the 'want to publish more'. I started looking at public health as a whole, and not as only the health of patients who came to my outpatient clinic or were admitted in my inpatient departments. Educating beyond the room was more satisfying than being that doctor who saw hundreds of patients a day without making a difference to the public.

I started taking up limited, but effective public-health-based research projects too, apart from my work-expertise-based studies. I stopped being the person married to my clinical work and research and stopped giving in to peer pressure and started understanding that nothing was more important than my own mental health, my family, wife and children. The work was there just enough to get my family going. Work was not everything.

In that process of compromise, I found time. And when I found time, I found things to do that made my family, and me, happy. The moment you learn to compromise, and find a path that leads you that way, life becomes beautiful.

Acknowledgements

I HAVE A SMALL BUT EXTREMELY IMPORTANT GROUP OF PEOPLE to acknowledge, thank and appreciate—the ones who helped me realize this book.

First, my patients. Where would I be without them? This is their book, not mine; these are their stories, which I have borrowed because they let me into their lives. For those I cared for, I remember you; and for those I care for now, I will never forget you; and for those awaiting my care, I will be there for you.

My Twitter friends (because it sounds weird to say X friends, no thanks to Elon) who read with patience and liked, loved and responded to my many long-form 'tweetorial' stories about my patients and their families, and shared them widely, made them viral. It is because of this that the book became a reality.

My wife, Teena, who let me write—enduring the deep loneliness of being with a husband who was present physically but whose mind was elsewhere. When I was exhausted, disturbed and just feeling low, she encouraged me to take baby steps and finish the marathon, rather than complete the sprint. I know she will not read this book, because all my stories are hers too and she already knows what this book holds.

My children—Alanna, Aideen and Arthur—who told me that I was working 'all the time' but still let me. I know they would have really wanted to spend more time with me, as the hospital became their first great rival and this book the second.

My parents and parents away from home, Cicy and Philip Augustine, and Cisamma and Johny George, respectively, who were as ecstatic as I was when they heard I was going to be an 'author'.

My brothers, Nebu, Ian and Lars; and sisters, Minna, Anushka and Amy; and my extended family of sisters and brothers—Maria and Tony, and Teny and Thomas—who promised me that this would be a life-changing experience. True to their words, it turned out to be the most demandingly poignant life-changing experience I have ever gone through.

My teachers Professor Prasanta Mukhopadhyay and Professor Partha Chattopadhyay, former head of department of medicine and former professor of medicine, respectively, at Nilratan Sircar Medical College and Hospital, Kolkata, West Bengal; and Professor Shiv Sarin, senior professor and head of department of hepatology and director of the Institute of Liver and Biliary Sciences, New Delhi—who not only taught me the art and craft of clinical medicine and hepatology, but also empathy, dedication and focus; and to listen more than speak, which helped me become the doctor my patients need me to be.

Last but not the least, and terrifically important, Ms Shabnam Srivastava, who sent me that first direct message on Twitter, asking me if I was interested in writing a book; Ms Bushra Ahmed of HarperCollins India; and the team who took it to the next level comfortably and without haste, the moment I said yes—for lending me a hand to get back the childhood I thought I had lost, and for finding me.

Appendix and Selected Bibliography

Scan this QR code to access the detailed notes.

About the Author

Dr Cyriac Abby Philips is a clinician-scientist in hepatology at Rajagiri Hospital, Kochi, Kerala. He completed his MBBS from St. Johns Medical College, Bengaluru; MD in internal medicine from Nil Ratan Sircar (NRS) Medical College, Kolkata; and DM in hepatology from the Institute of Liver and Biliary Sciences (ILBS), New Delhi. Under the viral handle 'The Liver Doc', he combats health misinformation across the Indian subcontinent, educating over 5 lakh followers on social media about liver health, as well as the dangers of pseudoscientific practices and alternative medicine. His data-driven, myth-busting posts, delivered with razor-edge sarcasm, have earned consistent national and international media coverage, making him India's most litigated science communicator. A prolific researcher and leading authority on herb- and supplement-induced liver injury, Dr Philips has been honoured with multiple awards from influential American, European, Asia-Pacific and Indian liver societies, including the Indian Society of Gastroenterology's Rising Star Award (2022) and the Indian Medical Association's coveted Social Media Award (2023). *The Liver Doctor* is his debut book.

About the Illustrator

My Lan (@LaolanArt) is a designer and illustrator based in the UK with a special love for book covers. She specializes in fantasy and romance, and strives to create meaningful and breathtaking illustrations. Her background in graphic design and concept art gives her flexibility in her illustration style and allows her to take a different approach to each project and make it unique. In her free time, she enjoys playing video games, reading and playing the bass guitar.

HarperCollins *Publishers* India

At HarperCollins India, we believe in telling the best stories and finding the widest readership for our books in every format possible. We started publishing in 1992; a great deal has changed since then, but what has remained constant is the passion with which our authors write their books, the love with which readers receive them, and the sheer joy and excitement that we as publishers feel in being a part of the publishing process.

Over the years, we've had the pleasure of publishing some of the finest writing from the subcontinent and around the world, including several award-winning titles and some of the biggest bestsellers in India's publishing history. But nothing has meant more to us than the fact that millions of people have read the books we published, and that somewhere, a book of ours might have made a difference.

As we look to the future, we go back to that one word—a word which has been a driving force for us all these years.

Read.

Harper Collins
Harper Sport
HARPER FICTION
HARPER NON-FICTION
हार्पर हिन्दी

HARPER LEARNING
HARPER VANTAGE
HCCB HARPERCOLLINS CHILDREN'S BOOKS
4th
HARPER PERENNIAL

HARPER DESIGN
BOOKTOPUS
HARPER BUSINESS